Ongoing Records Review

A Guide to The Joint Commission Compliance and Best Practice, Fifth Edition

Jean S. Clark, RHIA

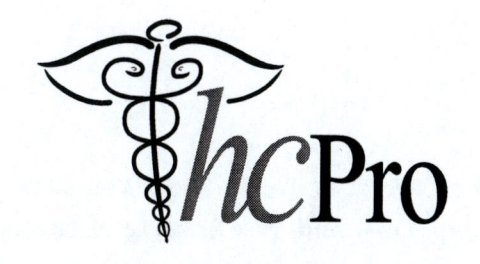

hcPro

Ongoing Records Review: A Guide to The Joint Commission Compliance and Best Practice, Fifth Edition is published by HCPro, Inc.

Copyright 2007, 2005, 2003, 2001, 1998 HCPro, Inc.

All rights reserved. Printed in the United States of America.   5   4   3   2   1

First edition published 1998. Second edition 2001. Third edition 2003. Fourth edition 2005. Fifth edition 2007

ISBN 978-1-57839-972-7

No part of this publication may be reproduced, in any form or by any means, without prior written consent of HCPro, Inc., or the Copyright Clearance Center (978/750-8400). Please notify us immediately if you have received an unauthorized copy.

HCPro, Inc., provides information resources for the healthcare industry.

HCPro, Inc. is not affiliated in any way with The Joint Commission, which owns the JCAHO and Joint Commission trademarks.

Jean S. Clark, RHIA, Author
Brian Murphy, Senior Managing Editor
Ilene G. MacDonald, Executive Editor
Lauren McLeod, Group Publisher
Mike Mirabello, Senior Graphic Artist
Jean St. Pierre, Director of Operations
Brenda Rossi, Cover Designer
Michael Roberto, Layout Artist

Advice given is general. Readers should consult professional counsel for specific legal, ethical, or clinical questions.

Arrangements can be made for quantity discounts. For more information, contact:

HCPro, Inc.
P.O. Box 1168
Marblehead, MA 01945
Telephone: 800/650-6787 or 781/639-1872
Fax: 781/639-2982
E-mail: *customerservice@hcpro.com*

Visit HCPro at its World Wide Web sites:
www.hcpro.com and www.hcmarketplace.com

02/2007
21100

Contents

List of figures v

About the author viii

Preface ix

    How this book is organized x
    How to install the CD-ROM xi

Chapter 1: Understanding ongoing records review
and The Joint Commission requirements 1

Chapter 2: Establishing an ongoing records review process 11

Chapter 3: Selecting review topics and indicators 19

Chapter 4: Using ongoing records review data to improve
medical records documentation 31

Chapter 5: Monitoring timeliness of records completion 35

Chapter 6: Demonstrating compliance to The Joint Commission surveyors 49

Chapter 7: Incorporating the tracer methodology
into ongoing records review 55

Contents

Chapter 8: Scoring and decision rules 75

Chapter 9: National Patient Safety Goals and other hot topics
for ongoing records review 81

Chapter 10: One hospital system's experience with two unannounced
Joint Commission surveys 109

Chapter 11: Case studies 133

Chapter 12: Sample review tools and reports 167

List of figures

Chapter One
Figure 1.1: Standard IM.6.10 5

Chapter Two
Figure 2.1: Ongoing records review process assessment 12
Figure 2.2: Ongoing records review oversight 14
Figure 2.3: Ongoing records review organization chart 18

Chapter Three
Figure 3.1: Admission history and physical examination 21
Figure 3.2: History and physical reports before surgery is performed 22
Figure 3.3: Ongoing review by provider 24
Figure 3.4: CABG clinical pathway 25
Figure 3.5: Emergency department ongoing records review calendar 28
Figure 3.6: Sample ongoing records review reporting calendar 29

Chapter Five
Figure 5.1: EPs related to timeliness and completion 36
Figure 5.2: 64 tips for improving timeliness of records completion 40

Chapter Six
Figure 6.1: A complete record 50
Figure 6.2: Delinquent records 50
Figure 6.3: Ongoing records review report 52
Figure 6.4: Quarterly summary report 53

Chapter Seven
Figure 7.1: Tracer case study 61
Figure 7.2: Patient tracer data collection form 63
Figure 7.3: Open/active chart review form 64

List of Figures

Figure 7.4: Priority focus audit form: Information management tracer .65
Figure 7.5: Patient tracer worksheet 67

Chapter Eight
Figure 8.1: The Joint Commission's levels of accreditation 78

Chapter Nine
Figure 9.1: Unapproved abbreviations audit day flier 84
Figure 9.2: Patient safety goals/documentation audit tool 85
Figure 9.3: Ongoing records review—open charts: Topic: Unapproved abbreviations 86
Figure 9.4: Sample unapproved abbreviations ongoing review tool 87
Figure 9.5: Universal Protocol for preventing wrong site,
          wrong procedure, wrong person surgery™ 90
Figure 9.6: Policy and procedure 92
Figure 9.7: Medication reconciliation form 94
Figure 9.8: Outpatient history and physical report 96
Figure 9.9: Postoperative progress note 98
Figure 9.10: Physician's preprinted orders 100
Figure 9.11: Sample legibility policy 101
Figure 9.12: Medical record review tool for pain management 105

Chapter Ten
Figure 10.1: The Joint Commission unannounced survey instruction sheet 112
Figure 10.2: Sample cover sheet for requested Joint Commission documents 113
Figure 10.3: Documents required for unannounced surveys 115
Figure 10.4: The Joint Commission check-off preparedness list 116
Figure 10.5: The Joint Commission sample survey questions 121
Figure 10.6: Departmental preparedness tips 125
Figure 10.7: The Joint Commission leadership interview reference sheet 129

Chapter Eleven
Figure 11.1: Sample open record review form 136
Figure 11.2: Progress note 139
Figure 11.3: Brief operative report 140
Figure 11.4: Day-of-surgery preprocedure note 141
Figure 11.5: Sample medical staff legibility policy 143
Figure 11.6: Sample open records review tool—adult inpatients 149
Figure 11.7: Ongoing documentation review tally sheet—Second quarter, 2005 154

Figure 11.8: Ongoing documentation review—Second quarter, 2005 159
Figure 11.9: Prohibited abbreviation documentation monitor 162
Figure 11.10: Prohibited abbreviation documentation tally 163
Figure 11.11: Action plan 164
Figure 11.12: Accountability letter 165

Chapter Twelve

Figure 12.1: Respiratory therapy chart review tool 169
Figure 12.2: Medical records documentation audit tool—physician office 170
Figure 12.3: Ongoing records review—inpatient records 171
Figure 12.4: Ongoing records review 172
Figure 12.5: Ongoing records review graph 173
Figure 12.6: Medical record deficiency trend compared to monthly discharges 174
Figure 12.7: First and second quarter comparison:
  Ongoing records review percentage met 175
Figure 12.8: Quarterly review summary 176
Figure 12.9: Ongoing records review—closed charts, discharge summary content 177

About the author

Jean S. Clark, RHIA

Jean S. Clark, RHIA, is the director of health information services at Roper Saint Francis Healthcare in Charleston, SC. She is a past president of the American Health Information Management Association (AHIMA) and the Quality Management Section of AHIMA and currently serves as the president of the International Federation of Health Records Organizations. Clark previously served as a member of The Joint Commission's Standards Review Task Force and the expert panel for the Information Management chapter. For six years, she was a member of The Joint Commission's Hospital Professional and Technical Advisory Committee. Clark also received AHIMA's Distinguished Member and Volunteer awards.

She is the author of *International Opportunities* from A *Career Guide for Health Information Management Professionals* (PRG Publishing, 1997), *Information Management: The Compliance Guide to the* JCAHO *Standards, Fifth Edition* (HCPro, 2004) and *Documentation Improvement Handbook for the Medical Staff* (HCPro, 2003). She is the contributing editor to *Medical Records Briefing*, published by HCPro, Inc. Clark is a frequent national and international speaker.

Preface

The year 2004 ushered in a new era for The Joint Commission, formerly known as the Joint Commission on Accreditation of Healthcare Organizations (JCAHO). A new process, fresh with revised standards and a revamped survey process, added value to accreditation and shifted the focus from "just in time" survey preparations to a continuous process of organizational improvement related to systems that affect patient care and safety. In addition to these changes, the standards related to ongoing review and completion of medical records underwent a facelift that should be a welcome change for providers.

In 2006, the era of The Joint Commission unannounced survey began. Hospitals and health information management (HIM) departments must now be on their toes for the unexpected arrival of survey teams. Year-round training and preparation are a must.

Despite these changes, some of the age-old questions remain: How does the organization perform ongoing records review in an effective and timely way, and how do you encourage physicians and other care providers to participate?

The revised standards and elements of performance (EPs) provide opportunities for innovation and change. Because their requirements are less prescriptive than in the past and because they provide greater flexibility in terms of what to review, organizations can turn what has often been a cumbersome paper-shuffling process into a streamlined ongoing records review process that really works.

Our goal in updating this practical guidebook is to give readers a clear explanation of the revised The Joint Commission requirements for ongoing records review and a step-by-step guide to developing a program that best suits the needs of your organization. This book breaks down the main elements of ongoing records review and provides samples of indicators and strategies that will lead to a successful process. Finally, it also includes the author's own unannounced survey experience and offers tips and best practices to help organizations prepare for an unannounced survey.

Preface

I hope this book will continue to provide you with a broader understanding of ongoing records review processes and practices and help you to take advantage of the opportunities for change afforded by the revised standards.

How this book is organized

Chapter 1 explains The Joint Commission's new accreditation process and requirements for ongoing records review.

In **Chapter 2**, you'll find information about how to establish an ongoing records review process at your organization.

Chapter 3 offers advice on how to select review topics and indicators.

Chapter 4 explains how your review teams and others report ongoing records review data, improve medical record documentation, and document results.

Chapter 5 explains why it's important to monitor the timeliness of records completion, as well as how to motivate physicians and gain the support of your administration and management.

In **Chapter 6**, we'll discuss the importance of the ongoing records review in The Joint Commission survey process and how to best demonstrate your program to surveyors.

Chapter 7 explains the importance of the medical record to The Joint Commission's new tracer methodology process and offers a case study on how you might conduct ongoing records review based on the tracer process.

Chapter 8 presents information on scoring and decision rules.

Chapter 9 discusses the importance of documentation and the National Patient Safety Goals. This chapter also includes advice about hot topics, such as legibility and delinquent records.

Chapter 10 presents one hospital system's experience with a pair of Joint Commission unannounced surveys and offers practical tips and advice for preparing for unannounced surveys.

In **Chapter 11**, you'll find several case studies that highlight different hospitals' successful programs.

Customizable sample forms and checklists are provided on the accompanying CD-ROM, including the 2006 medical record documentation guide. The CD-ROM also includes studies published in the third edition of this book. Although these case studies were developed before the 2004 standards, they represent good examples of the process needed to develop and sustain a successful ongoing records review program.

How to install the CD-ROM

This product was designed for the Windows operating system and includes Word files, which will run in Windows 95/98 or greater. The CD will work on all PCs and most Macintosh systems. To run the CD-ROM, take the following steps:

1. Insert the CD into your CD-ROM drive.
2. Double-click on the "My Computer" icon. Next, double-click on the CD-drive icon.
3. Double-click on the files you wish to open.
4. Adapt the files by moving the cursor over the areas you wish to change, highlighting them, and typing in the new information.
5. To save a file to your facility's system, click on "File" and then click on "Save As." Select the location where you wish to save the file, and then click on "Save."
6. To print a document, click on "File" and then click on "Print."

CHAPTER 1

Understanding ongoing records review and The Joint Commission requirements

Introduction: New standards, new accreditation process

In 2001, The Joint Commission established the standards review task force. Its primary goal was to provide a new accreditation process that would focus on systems critical to safe, quality care, so it asked representatives from healthcare organizations across the country to review the hospital accreditation standards, scoring, and survey process. The task force's work resulted in The Joint Commission's establishment of a new era in accreditation that began in January 2004: Shared Visions–New Pathways®.

This new process incorporates an annual self-assessment called the "periodic performance review" (PPR), in which organizations determine their compliance with the standards. Organizations also experience an on-site survey tailored to their priority focus processes (PFPs) or the types of services they provide. During the survey, instead of visiting every nursing unit and support department, the surveyors use "tracer methodology" to follow patients through the organization. This approach requires surveyors to interview staff in various units about the specific care of the patient being traced.

Scoring, accreditation decisions, and reporting have also changed with the revised standards. In 2006, The Joint Commission began conducting unannounced, on-site surveys, thereby increasing the need for hospitals to be continuously in compliance with standards and avoid the rush to "get things in order" immediately prior to their survey dates.

As part of the new accreditation process, The Joint Commission has deleted, revised, or incorporated into different chapters many of its standards. Ultimately, there will be one accreditation manual that serves all types of organizations. But for now, hospitals rely on the revised *Comprehensive Accreditation Manual for Hospitals* (CAMH), which includes the following chapters:

Chapter One

Patient-focused functions:
- Ethics, rights, and responsibilities (RI)
- Provision of care, treatment, and services (PC)
- Medication management (MM)
- Surveillance, prevention, and control of infection (IC)

Organizational functions:
- Improving organization performance (PI)
- Leadership (LD)
- Management of the environment of care (EC)
- Management of human resources (HR)
- Management of information (IM)

Structures with functions:
- Medical staff (MS)
- Nursing (NR)

The format of the chapters has changed, offering organizations a better understanding of The Joint Commission's expectations for compliance with each standard. This new format includes the following:

- The standard, which defines the performance expectations, structures, or processes that must be in place for an organization to provide safe and high-quality care, treatment, and service.

- The rationale for, background on, justification for, and additional information about a standard. The rationale is not scored, and not every standard has a rationale.

- The element of performance (EP), which describes the specific performance expectations/ structures or processes that must be in place to provide safe, high-quality care, treatment, and services. The EPs are scored to determine accreditation compliance.

Each EP under a standard—and any associated bullets—are scored based upon categories A, B, or C:

- Category A EPs are based upon the presence or absence of the requirements and are scored either "yes" or "no."

Understanding ongoing records review and The Joint Commission requirements

- Category B EPs are based upon the presence or absence of the requirement, as well as compliance with the principles of good process design.

- Category C EPs are scored based upon the number of times an EP is not met. Category C EPs require a measure of success (MOS) to validate compliance.

It is important to understand the scoring methodology when you conduct your PPRs and your ongoing records review. A clear understanding of the scoring will provide a clear picture of your organization's compliance and readiness for survey.

The new ongoing records review requirements

As part of the new accreditation process, you'll see different requirements for ongoing records review. For example, the standard is no longer a standard—it has become EPs 12 and 13 under standard IM.6.10. The good news about this is that you are no longer required to review the 19 items spelled out under the old standards. A few requirements remain the same, however:

- **Ongoing records review**—This requirement now has a less prescriptive approach, which provides greater leeway in developing individual records review processes.

- **Point-of-care reviews**—The Joint Commission continues to emphasize open records reviews over closed records reviews (which occur after discharge). In fact, The Joint Commission no longer even mentions closed chart reviews. Part of the reason is that point-of-care reviews enable you to correct documentation issues while the patient is being treated. Most standards continue to be time-sensitive before discharge, not after.

- **PI approach**—Although not required by IM.6.10, EPs 12 and 13, a PI approach should continue to be the foundation of records review. As with any PI activity, data should be aggregated and analyzed to identify trends and opportunities for improvement in this process. Whenever possible, conduct a root-cause analysis to determine action plans and identify the focus of future reviews and follow-up. Variations in records review primarily result from flawed processes, so you will rarely have to look at individuals; nevertheless, there may be times when an individual staff member, physician, or department will be the focus of your action plan. As a reminder, the EPs do not require the review of records for every physician on your staff.

Chapter One

The new records review requirement (IM.6.10, EPs 12 and 13) provides flexibility for the individual facility to develop a systematic and effective approach to identifying opportunities for improvement related to the medical record. Even with this flexibility, however, remember that the medical record serves as the foundation for patient care and safety, so it only makes sense to ensure that it is accurate, complete, and timely.

Organizations now have an even greater choice than they did before about how often they conduct medical records reviews and what indicators and methodology they use. These changes will ultimately make the records review process more effective, efficient, and meaningful.

The health information management (HIM) director will continue to play an important role in the process as facilitator, educator, and information source. In fact, as the following chapters will show, the revised standards provide more opportunity for the HIM director to serve as a facilitator rather than the person who must perform the less than gratifying task of reviewing closed records.

How this book will help

Understanding The Joint Commission's new records review EPs is the foundation of an effective ongoing records review program, so this first chapter details the EPs and their requirements for compliance. However, because The Joint Commission's new EPs are only a starting point in understanding ongoing records review, the remaining chapters of the book detail the essential activities of and decisions involved in setting up such a program.

The standard and EPs explained

The new EPs are a lot to consider. Although they are prescriptive in some ways, they still allow for flexibility that the standards of the past did not. They do indicate that organizations must have an ongoing review process at the point of care (i.e., the time that the patient is in the hospital or being treated in an outpatient setting). These records are sometimes referred to as "open records," as opposed to "closed records," which are associated with patients who have been discharged or have completed treatment.

Organizations can use computer applications, such as the HIM analysis/incomplete record systems, to provide target areas for point-of-care reviews.

Figure 1.1

Standard IM.6.10

Standard IM.6.10

The hospital has complete and accurate medical records for patients assessed, cared for, treated, or served.

Rationale for IM.6.10

Patient-specific data and information are contained in the medical record, both inpatient and outpatient, to facilitate patient care, treatment, and services; serve as a financial and legal record; aid in research; support decision analysis; and guide professional and organizational performance improvement. This information may be maintained as a paper record or as electronic health information.

Element of Performance 12

Medical records are reviewed on an ongoing basis at the point of care.

Element of Performance 13

The review of medical records is based on hospital-defined indicators that address the presence, timeliness, readability (whether handwritten or printed), quality, consistency, clarity, accuracy, completeness, and authentication of data and information contained within the record.

Source: www.jointcommission.org; 2006 Comprehensive Accreditation Manual for Hospitals, "Management of Information" chapter, Oakbrook Terrace, IL: The Joint Commission.

Chapter One

Your organization can define its own indicators, although it must address at some point (but not in every review) the following attributes:

- *Presence of data and information*—Is the required data available?

    For example, is the history and physical (H&P) on the paper record or available electronically?

- *Timeliness*—Are documents available according to standards, organization policy, and state or federal laws? Is care provided to the patient in the most beneficial way and within the necessary time frame?

    For example, is the H&P report on the chart or available electronically within 24 hours of admission to the hospital?

- *Readability* (whether handwritten or printed)—Are the entries legible and easy to read?

    For example, is the handwritten H&P legible and understandable? Are copies of reports legible and free of obstructive marks?

- *Quality*—Does the documentation reflect an accurate picture of the care and treatment provided? Is it meaningful and appropriate to the encounter?

    For example, does the H&P contain all the items required by hospital policy and additional information relevant to the condition for which the patient is being treated?

- *Consistency*—Does the medical record consistently reflect good standards of documentation practices and principles? Are the forms or computer screens standardized?

    For example, all paper forms are required to have the patient label on the top right-hand corner and the name of the organization on the top left. All forms must be identified as to their purpose. The menus for charting must be consistent for all types of data entry.

- *Clarity*—Is the meaning of each entry clear?

For example, do all orders for medications contain who gave the order, who received and recorded the order, the type of medication, the dosage, and the time period in which to administer the medication?

- *Accuracy*—Are entries free from error and in accord with documentation guidelines?

   For example, are all transcribed reports free of blanks?

- *Completeness*—Does the medical record contain all the reports and documentation to support the treatment provided?

   For example, is the medical record complete according to policy and the care that was given?

- *Authentication*—Has the medical record been validated for correctness, both for the information itself and for the person who is the author or user of the information?

   For example, at the time of discharge, has the record been analyzed for appropriate reports and signatures?

Perhaps you think the 19 items formerly mandated by The Joint Commission for records review were easier to handle, as was that long tool used by surveyors for open and closed records review. There's no doubt you will need some time to get comfortable with the new EPs. However, the EPs will provide a pathway to more accurate, timely, and complete medical records in a simplified process for reviews that will result in better patient care and safety for patients.

Even though the EPs don't mention who should participate and report in the ongoing records review, it is important to involve in the process the people who document in the record. In fact, they still need to be the reviewers, but you can simplify the process to focus on areas that most need improvement.

Sample size

The standard and EPs do not identify a sample size, but The Joint Commission has defined sample sizes when monitoring compliance with category C EPs. They are

- all cases for a population size of fewer than 30

Chapter One

- 30 cases for a population size of 30–100
- 50 cases for a population size of 101–500
- 70 cases for a population size of more than 500

You can use these guides for ongoing records review as well.

Records completion statistics

There are EPs under IM.6.10 that require organizations to define a complete record and measure medical record delinquency at regular intervals. Many facilities monitor records completion through a process separate from their ongoing records review. See Chapter 5 for a discussion of how to monitor records completion and delinquency.

Important decisions and activities of ongoing records review

Although the previous section summarizes the contents of The Joint Commission's standard and EPs for ongoing records review, it will take more than just an understanding of the standard to comply with The Joint Commission's requirements and establish an effective ongoing records review program. Successful ongoing records review continues to require well-planned, well-executed activities. Now, however, organizations can select what works best for them.

In planning your ongoing records review program, your facility must make the following decisions:

- What indicators will we use to measure compliance with IM.6.10, EPs 12 and 13?

- How often will we carry out ongoing records review (e.g., weekly, monthly, as issues arise)?

- Who will review the records?

- How will we identify PI opportunities?

- How and by whom will ongoing records review data be aggregated and summarized into meaningful information?

Understanding ongoing records review and The Joint Commission requirements

- How will we gather representative samples of records?

- How, how often, and to whom will ongoing records review findings be presented?

- How will we document ongoing records review activities, actions, and improvements for Joint Commission PPRs and on-site surveys?

The following chapters will answer these questions and provide examples to assist you with your own review process. Organizations also must coordinate the above decisions with the planning and execution of the following activities:

- **Training** individuals responsible for records review

- **Gathering** representative samples (if appropriate) of medical records for review

- **Analyzing** items in medical records against the established records review indicators

- **Presenting** data to the group responsible for oversight of ongoing records review

- **Reporting** ongoing records review–related findings to appropriate individuals, committees, departments, and other groups

- **Planning** and carrying out PI activities to improve medical records documentation, based upon ongoing records review findings

- **Documenting** actions and improvements related to ongoing records review

Because The Joint Commission provides little guidance in the EPs on how to plan and execute the ongoing records review, facilities must develop programs that meet their particular organizational needs—they must make the above decisions and plan the above activities themselves.

CHAPTER 2

Establishing an ongoing records review process

Introduction

As discussed in Chapter 1, The Joint Commission's ongoing records review standard and elements of performance (EPs) outline specific requirements for records review, but they are far less detailed than the accreditor's previous records review standards.

The Joint Commission's intent is to provide organizations with flexibility in developing a process that best suits their needs. Thus, each organization has broad discretion in deciding the who, what, when, and how of ongoing records review. The danger posed by this flexibility, however, is that it could result in a less effective process.

This chapter will provide guidance on redesigning your process to achieve accurate, timely, and complete medical records.

To change or not to change

Just because the requirements have changed does not mean you have to totally redo your process. Conducting a simple assessment will help your organization identify ways to improve and simplify its process in view of the flexibility now afforded by the standard and the EPs. Figure 2.1 provides a few questions your organization should ask before you decide how to change your process.

Figure 2.1

Ongoing records review process assessment

Question	Examples	Comments/actions
1. What works?		
2. What does not work?		
3. Is the structure right for the current requirements and the organization?		
4. Is there an easier way to collect information from existing processes/systems?		
5. What, if any, meaningful changes have occurred as a result of the ongoing records review process?		
6. Should we automate the process? What is available?		

Components of a records review process

A good records review process still consists of the following five major steps:

1. Decide what to review, who will conduct the reviews, and how often to conduct reviews
2. Review the records
3. Collect and organize the data
4. Analyze the data and take action
5. Assemble an oversight team specifically for ongoing records review

This review process usually involves the following three groups of professionals:

- The individuals actually reviewing the records
- The support staff who organize the data
- The group (or individual) who oversees the overall ongoing records review program

An existing team or committee provides all or a portion of the five major components of the process. Whatever the structure is, someone needs to take the lead, become the expert in the requirements, and begin the process of revitalizing the organization's ongoing records review program.

1. Decide what to review, who will conduct the reviews, and how often to conduct reviews

Because many healthcare facility activities require interdisciplinary review teams, an organization may find that an existing group, team, or committee is well-suited to oversee ongoing records review. The medical records committee, if one exists in the organization, is already familiar with medical records and performs activities similar to ongoing records review, such as analyzing medical records for completeness and timeliness. Figure 2.2 illustrates a protocol for a medical record committee with ongoing records review oversight, but you should modify the example for whatever group is charged with this responsibility.

In smaller organizations, the PI or medical executive committee can serve as the oversight group. Such a group generally does not review records but rather coordinates the process by helping to establish indicators, deciding how often reviews will occur, receiving and analyzing reports, and deciding what focused reviews the organization should carry out.

The organization's leadership must decide who selects the topics and indicators for review (i.e., the oversight group or the departments), who will collect the information, and how often departments will report to the oversight group. The most successful approach would be to have the oversight group and the departments agree on review topics and indicators or focused reviews based on previous data related to ongoing records review. See Chapter 3 for more about selecting topics and indicators.

Figure 2.2

Ongoing records review oversight protocol

Purpose
The medical records committee will have oversight for the organization's ongoing records review program and the review and approval of forms and format for the medical record.

Scope
All types of medical records and related functions, including paper-based and electronic will be encompassed.

Responsibilities
Coordination and oversight of the organization's ongoing records review program, including
- establishing the calendar for reviews
- assisting with topic and indicator selection
- establishing focused reviews
- analyzing data from reviews, and taking actions as appropriate
- conducting point-of-care reviews using the tracer methodology
- reporting to appropriate organization and medical staff committees
- reviewing and approving of forms and format for the medical record, including electronic applications
- reviewing of the monthly delinquent record statistics and taking action as needed
- performing other duties as they relate to the documentation, use, and storage of medical records

Membership
Membership will include physicians, nurses, other clinical care providers, HIM managers, and others as identified by the committee. A physician in good standing on the medical staff will chair the committee.

Meetings
Meetings will occur monthly on the first Tuesday of each month at 7:00 a.m.

Reporting
Departments and nursing units will report bimonthly (based upon a schedule published in January of each year). The committee will report quarterly to the PI council and the medical executive committee.

Statement of confidentiality
Members of the committee will honor patients' rights to privacy with respect to information in the medical records. All reports will be free of patient identifiers.

2. Review the records

Actual reviews of the medical records should occur at the point of care by the individuals who either document in the records or enter data into the electronic record. Note that health information management (HIM) department staff (i.e., coders, record analysts, and managers) can assist with any retrospective reviews that may be necessary and, ideally, will review records for completeness, authentication, and quality of discharge summaries. They also can serve as backup reviewers for unapproved abbreviations and legibility. See Chapter 9 for more information of reviews related to unapproved abbreviations and other National Patient Safety Goals issues. See Chapter 11 for a case study about a successful legibility review.

Because most Joint Commission standards and EPs are time-sensitive (i.e., they apply while the patient is being treated), reviews of closed records are less productive than point-of-care reviews.

3. Collect and organize data

This function is ideally suited to the HIM or performance improvement (PI) director, both of whom are skilled at aggregating, displaying, and analyzing data and information. Ideally the record reviewers enter their findings into a computer software program that is networked throughout the organization. Then collecting and organizing data become a simple matter of running reports for the oversight group and the departments conducting the reviews. There are software applications on the market, as well as "home grown" systems, that can make data collection and report generation much easier. See Chapter 11 for case studies of various hospitals' successes with these types of tools.

If your organization still uses paper for this process, have the reviews come to a centralized location so they can be organized and reports can be generated.

4. Analyze the data and take action

The oversight group generally analyzes data and takes appropriate action, but because each department that conducts reviews can receive task assignments, be sure to establish and adhere to a schedule for reporting to the oversight group. Such a well-structured process will help emphasize the importance of ongoing records review and stress to all involved that they should not take this process lightly.

5. Assemble an oversight team specifically for ongoing records review

Although some organizations use established committees or combine the ongoing records review oversight function with other reviews, other organizations choose to create an interdisciplinary team

Chapter Two

dedicated to ongoing records review. The latter approach may help draw attention to the importance of ongoing records review and may help a facility assemble a group of professionals who are interested in and committed to the process. See Chapter 7 for a team approach to ongoing records review using the tracer methodology.

Note that, to be successful, the interdisciplinary team should have the authority to make improvements. In addition, team members must understand the review process and motivate the organization to effect change.

Select the facilitator
Regardless of how an organization chooses to structure its actual review process, make sure that the facilitator for the ongoing records review process is not also the chair of the oversight team. The HIM director or someone from the HIM department is a good candidate for this position. Such candidates will be familiar with the content of medical records and the resources for topics and indicators—and, more important, are experts in database management and data display. Another good candidate for the facilitator position is the PI director, who is also familiar with the use of data and PI methodologies.

Select physicians to be team members
Include on the team physicians who are willing and able to champion the cause of good documentation. Such physicians should have the respect of their peers and be interested in and understand the importance of good documentation.

Try selecting candidates from former members of the medical record and PI committees. The vice president of medical affairs and past medical staff presidents are also good choices for leaders or team members.

Select nurses and other clinical professionals to be team members
The selection of nurses and other clinical professionals is equally important. Choose individuals who are interested in the ongoing records review process and, ideally, have been involved in developing either forms for their particular specialties or computer applications for electronic charting. Staff who have served on a clinical pathway team, as utilization reviewers, or as PI coordinators make excellent candidates; they are familiar with reviewing records based upon set indicators, regardless of whether the oversight team conducts actual records reviews.

The chief nurse executive (CNE) is essential to a successful ongoing records review program. Because nurses are usually the ones who perform point-of-care reviews, the CNE's support is vital, so he or she should always be a member of the oversight team. To make that happen, "sell" the CNE on the importance of timely, accurate, and complete documentation to the new survey process and on the fact that nursing staff will be on the frontlines at the time of survey. See Chapter 7 for an example of an ongoing records review approach using the tracer methodology that CNEs have applied successfully.

Select other team members

Although The Joint Commission's new EPs don't address how the ongoing records review team should be organized, be sure that it includes other caregivers who document in the medical record. Support staff, such as admitting office staff, coders, and information technology managers, can round out the team.

Orientation and training

Once you've selected the process, team configuration, and participants, provide adequate orientation and training of all those involved in ongoing records review. Establish orientation and periodic refresher courses in records review methodology, the selection of indicators, and the analysis and reporting of data. See Chapter 11 for an explanation of how one organization used technology to orient and train its staff about ongoing records review.

Efficient ongoing records review practices

When planning the ongoing records review process, an organization has to consider the schedules of many people—most of whom have limited time and multiple commitments—especially if the team members conduct the actual review. If they do, then select a time each month to conduct reviews. Choose a meeting place either in the units/departments or in a central location where records can be brought to the team.

The latter approach, however, often is not practical, because staff need records for patient care. Therefore, an alternative would be to assign team members to units/departments and allow them to review records at the points of care at their convenience. The simplest and best approach to conducting the actual reviews is to have designated staff on each unit/department conduct their own reviews and report their findings to the oversight team. Figure 2.3 illustrates an example of an ongoing records review organization chart.

CHAPTER TWO

Figure 2.3

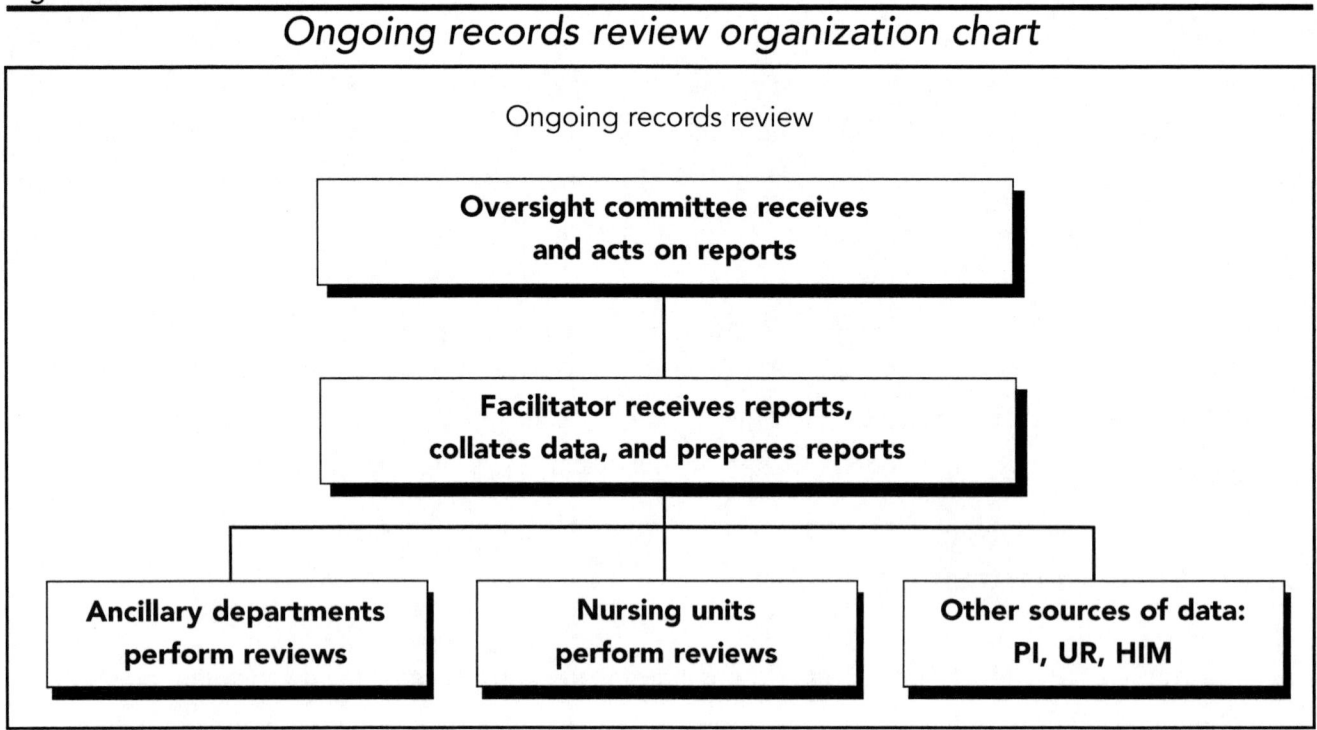

Ongoing records review organization chart

Ongoing records review

- Oversight committee receives and acts on reports
- Facilitator receives reports, collates data, and prepares reports
  - Ancillary departments perform reviews
  - Nursing units perform reviews
  - Other sources of data: PI, UR, HIM

Note that you can incorporate records review into existing activities, such as utilization review, clinical pathway processes, and PI. Because these functions are already in place, they are good sources for gathering information for focused reviews.

Reporting the findings

Regardless of the organization's process, periodically (e.g., quarterly or semiannually) report the results of the ongoing records review to the leadership of the organization and the medical staff.

Chapter 3

Selecting review topics and indicators

Because The Joint Commission has modified its standards related to ongoing records review, selecting the topics and indicators may seem like the most difficult task in revising the process.

Samples

Although a sample size is not mentioned in IM.6.10, elements of performance (EPs) 12 and 13, be sure to review enough records that you can establish trends over time. Such review will allow you to aggregate data and identify where you need to focus future studies to ensure continuous compliance (which is important for patient care and safety) and help you complete the annual periodic performance review (PPR) and prepare for unannounced surveys. Additionally, if you are not in compliance with an EP, you must develop a corrective action plan. Because so many EPs throughout the *Comprehensive Accreditation Manual for Hospitals* are still based upon documentation in the medical records, an effective ongoing records review program is essential.

When selecting samples (e.g., the number or type of records to review), do what works best for your organization. For example, if the hospital has 25 obstetrical patients a year and decides to include these types of patients in its ongoing records review, then it should review all 25 cases. Conduct these reviews as the patients are admitted and develop specific indicators based upon hospital-defined criteria.

Another approach might be to consider your annual admissions. Basing the number of records to review in your sample upon that number and spreading the reviews throughout the year reduces the number of records that are being reviewed at any one time. Just remember to include all the services you provide at some (or several) points in your program—don't forget the ambulatory areas, especially physician office practices owned by the organization. See Chapter 1 for information on sample sizes.

CHAPTER THREE

Topics and indicators

The primary goal of the review process is to ensure the quality of medical records for all patients. Therefore, your organization must select topics and indicators for ongoing reviews that are appropriate for the organization. Although review teams or committees are ultimately responsible for selecting sample records and indicators, this chapter suggests how to involve other groups in these processes.

Because the sample size, indicators, and responsibilities of ongoing reviews can vary widely among organizations, and because there are many ways of complying with The Joint Commission standards, this chapter will discuss only the main issues that organizations need to consider when structuring their own programs.

Getting started: Using available data to focus reviews

A good way to start is to consider what data you already have. Organizations have been performing record reviews for a long time, so use your past data to determine how to focus your reviews. Prior to The Joint Commission's 2004 revisions, organizations spent so much time collecting data on so many indicators that they did not have time to focus on problems. Now, however, the opportunity exists to reduce the number of items reviewed and focus on the documentation issues that continue to be problematic.

Data is available from many sources, such as incomplete-record analysis systems, performance improvement (PI), and utilization review. Figure 3.1 illustrates how the organization could conduct a focused review of history and physical (H&P) examinations at the point of care using retrospective data from the medical record analysis system. For example, the past three months' incomplete-record analysis indicates that the departments of surgery, obstetrics, and orthopedics have the greatest numbers of records deficient for H&Ps after discharge. To conduct a review focused on that issue at the point of care, use the tool from Figure 3.1, which includes some of the requirements from EP 13. Targeted areas of the organization would participate, and some of the indicators required in the new EP 13 would be used to review the records.

Figure 3.1

Admission history and physical examination

Indicator	Addresses	Met	Not met	Comments
1. H&P charted or available electronically within 24 hrs. of admission	Presence; timeliness			
2. Handwritten H&P is legible	Readability			
3. Transcribed H&P is accurate, no blanks	Accuracy			
4. The H&P includes, at minimum, assessment of the heart, lungs, and condition for which the patient is being admitted	Quality			
5. Within 30 days after discharge, the H&P is authenticated by the appropriate MD	Authentication			

Items 1–4 are reviewed concurrently; Item 5 is reviewed by HIM staff checking the H&P in the transcription system because the medical staff rules and regulations allow this time frame for the authentication of H&Ps.

Another example of using a focused-review approach that measures the presence, timeliness, and quality of H&Ps prior to surgery is illustrated in Figure 3.2. Past records review data indicates that H&P reports were not on the medical record before surgery and that the records did not contain the minimum information for H&Ps required by the medical staff rules and regulations.

Thus, the organization decided to conduct a focused review of records prior to surgery in the same-day surgery department. In this review, the nursing staff use a simple check-off form for one month

Figure 3.2

History and physical reports before surgery is performed

Are the following critical elements present?

Indicator	Yes	No	Comments
Is the H&P on the chart prior to surgery? If yes, continue (**presence and timeliness**)			
Content includes:			
Heart exam (**quality**)			
Lung exam (**quality**)			
Mental status (**quality**)			
Exam of body system relative to procedure (**quality**)			

to review all surgery patients (see Figure 3.2). The form remains in the medical record, and at discharge, the health information management (HIM) staff enter the findings in a database. The organization then presents aggregate findings from the focused review to the surgery department for analysis, action, and reporting to the coordinating committee.

Postoperative progress notes and telephone orders are other medical staff focused-review topics because these often remain challenges for a timely and complete medical record. You can extract the baseline data from the record analysis system.

Although these two examples have focused on the medical staff, previous ongoing records review data, PI, and other clinical benchmarking data can provide topics for focused reviews for other caregivers.

Starting over

If you want to simply start over, this is the time to do it. Conduct the assessment outlined in Chapter 2, and determine what has and hasn't worked in the past. Your organization can use this information to decide how to refocus its ongoing records review process, and because The Joint Commission offers organizations flexibility in which review topics they select, the sky is the limit. Start by categorizing records by potential topics, such as

- diagnostic-related groups (DRGs)

- diagnosis

- department (e.g., obstetrics, surgical, emergency, ambulatory surgery)

- sections of the medical record (e.g., assessments, plans of care, orders, operative and anesthesia, restraints)

- categories defined in The Joint Commission's EPs (e.g., presence, timeliness, readability, etc.)

- care providers

Also ask departments to select their own topics and indicators. The HIM and PI departments can help with data analysis to determine where you should focus the ongoing process. Figure 3.3 provides an example of how an organization might select topics for review based upon care providers and using baseline data from available sources to identify focused reviews.

You could develop this provider review further to include dietitians, respiratory therapists, and other caregivers within the organization. Chapter 11 provides a case study on one hospital's decision to "start over" with its ongoing record review process.

Review at the point of care (open records)

Caregivers who document in the record should perform ongoing reviews at the point of care. If possible, use simple check forms or, better yet, handheld devices or intranet applications to enter findings. The CD-ROM provides a case study example of how one hospital developed its own intranet application for collecting data for the ongoing records review process.

Figure 3.3

Ongoing review by provider

Provider	Topic(s)	Indicator
Medical staff	H&P prior to surgery (include inpatient and outpatient records)	• Present before surgery • Contains past history; exam of heart, lungs; review of systems pertinent to procedure
Nursing	Initial assessment (all inpatient units and ED)	• Present within 24 hrs. of admission or one hour in ED • No blanks on form • Pain assessed with a numerical score • Authenticated
Physical therapy (PT)	Assessments (inpatients)	• Responded to referral within 48 hrs. • Care plan includes PT goals based upon assessment

Other sources of data

As mentioned previously, use as much data and information from other sources of chart reviews as possible. Do not reinvent the wheel if someone else is already gathering data.

For example, you can use clinical paths as review tools, either to identify documentation problems or to monitor documentation. You could add indicators, such as those noted in Figures 3.2 and 3.3, to the path form, and a nurse could check them off as part of the daily path review. Because documentation is a key component of a critical path, the path is often a great tool to identify documentation

Figure 3.4

CABG clinical pathway

Process to improve	Timing of daily weights and lab specimen collection for postop CABG patients
Team	CABG clinical path team
Problem statement	Department director had 10 patient complaints last month stating that they could not get any rest while in the hospital and were awakened before daylight to be weighed and have lab work done.
Sources of variations	• Surgeons must make rounds between 6 a.m. and 7 a.m., as surgical cases start at 7 a.m. The lab results need to be on the chart consistently by 7 a.m.
	• The lab reports that 40% of its workload occurs between 5 a.m. and 8 a.m. Many a.m. labs are ordered as "STAT" on a routine basis, which backlogs orders of truly STAT orders.
	• Patients say that they cannot get back to sleep after the 5 a.m. wake-up.
	Literature review suggests that timing of weights and routine labs for CABG patients need to be consistent from one 24-hour period to the next for trending; however, there is no clinical significance regarding what time of the day the measurements should be obtained.

opportunities. Figure 3.4 illustrates a PI opportunity identified using a coronary artery bypass graft (CABG) path.

Figure 3.4 illustrates data that the organization was already monitoring and that addressed timeliness in regard to a DRG. Other good sources of data, either to incorporate as part of your reviews or to use to determine where you should focus, include the following:

CHAPTER THREE

Figure 3.4 (cont.)

CABG clinical pathway

Plan improvement	• Physicians order daily weights and routine lab work for 9 p.m.
	• Protocol for routine weights and routine lab collection to be changed from 5 a.m. to 9 p.m.
	• Monitor patient and physician complaints for a 60-day trial period. Monitor incidence of lab results on chart by 6 a.m.
Do	January 1
Check	Analysis on March 15 revealed no patient complaints regarding sleep disturbance for weight and labs. No physician complaints regarding absence of lab work on charts for a.m. rounds. Monitoring revealed that 100% of routine labs ordered were on the charts at 6 a.m.
Act	Continue with 9 p.m. weights and routine lab collection time for CABG patients.

- Core measure data
- State or national databases to which you submit data (e.g., the National Perinatal Database)
- PI teams

Note that trying to document Medicare's core measure data has been challenging for some hospitals. One hospital decided to make this documentation part of its ongoing records review and, in doing so, has been successful in raising its compliance rates and awareness of the need to document these important aspects of patient care.

As this chapter illustrates, many sources can generate ongoing records review topic ideas. As stated before, you can select topics based on findings from generic criteria on a random sample of records, recommendations of other committees or teams, known documentation problems, frequent diagnoses and procedures, and hospital statistical reports. The organization must identify what is useful to its programs and services while continuing to meet The Joint Commission standards and EPs for documentation in the medical record and ongoing medical records review.

Documentation requirements for the medical record

This book does not encourage reverting to the multiple-page tool organizations used in the past, but it does include a line-by-line description of the standards and EPs related to documentation requirements in the medical record (see the 2006 medical records documentation guide on the accompanying CD-ROM). Although you can use this guide to select topics for record reviews, don't fall into the trap of looking at everything all the time.

A planned approach

Whatever your methodology for selecting topics for review and developing indicators to meet the EPs, a planned approach is essential to a useful process. Just checking off the items on tools used in the past is not the most effective way to perform ongoing records review. Rather, the best approach is to get the people who document in the medical record (whether paper or electronic) to decide what is important to measure to ensure timely, accurate, and complete medical records. Nevertheless, for best results, always keep it simple. Figure 3.5 illustrates how the emergency department might set up its review of records for a 12-month period.

Good planning and direction for participants in the ongoing records review process is essential. When departments know what is expected of them, they will get the job done in an efficient and effective manner. Therefore, the oversight committee should develop a reporting calendar and distribute it at the beginning of each year to all departments participating in the process. Departments can select their own reviews and establish their own indicators, but the oversight committee also can request focused reviews at various times throughout the year. Figure 3.6 illustrates an organization's 12-month plan for reporting ongoing review activities.

The calendar in Figure 3.6 is an example of a planned approach to ongoing records review. In it, each department identifies its own indicators, either by analysis of previous data or at the direction of the facilitator or oversight committee. The departments review the records and enter data into an electronic system or onto worksheets. Then the HIM or PI department collects data for the medical staff

Figure 3.5

Emergency department ongoing records review calendar

Topic	Jan	Feb	Mar	Apr	May	Jun	Jul	Aug	Sep	Oct	Nov	Dec
Nursing:												
Initial assessment	X			X			X			X		
Pain management		X			X			X			X	
Authentication and readability			X			X			X			X
Medical staff:												
H&P	X			X			X			X		
Transfers		X			X			X			X	
Discharge instructions			X			X			X			X
Nursing/medical staff:												
Use of restraints												
Use of moderate sedation												

and provides focused topics to be incorporated into the point-of-care reviews performed by nursing/ other appropriate departments. The oversight committee conducts two reviews per year using the tracer methodology, and the coordinating committee receives the resulting reports. If they have indicators that are not compliant for two reporting periods, departments attend the committee meeting.

One organization's process for conducting review may not work for another. That's the beauty of the revised EP—one size does not fit all. So even though you must ensure that your records review program includes certain basic elements, experiment to create the most efficient and effective program. And don't forget to make it simple for everyone involved.

Figure 3.6

Sample ongoing records review reporting calendar

Department	Jan	Feb	Mar	Apr	May	Jun	Jul	Aug	Sep	Oct	Nov	Dec
Medical staff depts.				x				x				x
Nursing units		x				x				x		
Emergency depts.			x				x				x	
Support depts.; for example, PT, lab, radiology	x				x				x			
ORs and outpatient surgery			x				x				x	
Clinics	x				x				x			
HIM dept. abbreviations, discharge summary, delinquent rates				x				x				x
Tracer methodology mock surveys	x						x					
Other		x				x				x		

CHAPTER 4

Using ongoing records review data to improve medical records documentation

Regardless of who does the initial review of medical records in an ongoing review program, the oversight committee/departments are responsible for reviewing the data and either acting on the findings or recommending actions for others to take. As mentioned in Chapter 2, it's useful to designate an individual as the facilitator for the overall program so he or she can act as the contact for the following tasks:

- Developing review tools
- Carrying out education and training
- Providing a repository for the collected data
- Aggregating and displaying the findings
- Preparing reports for the oversight group and for the departments that perform the reviews

Control charts, graphs, and other performance improvement (PI) tools will enhance the review of the information and enable departments to come to quick conclusions about what actions to take. This chapter considers how review teams and others report information, implement improvements, and document results. See Chapter 6 for a discussion of the importance of this documentation in The Joint Commission's survey process.

Reporting initial findings and identifying problem records

Those responsible for reviewing records and gathering data should submit reports that include, at a minimum, the following information:

- The types of records reviewed
- The time period during which the information was gathered
- The total number of records reviewed
- The number of records found in compliance (or not in compliance) with the criteria
- Descriptions of problems uncovered, if applicable

Chapter Four

If you use a computer application, reviewers must evaluate the records and data entry. The facilitator then collects the data and prepares reports that include the above information. To make the data more meaningful, staff who collect the data and prepare the reports should note the percentages of records reviewed and found in compliance with criteria. For example, learning that 85% of records were in compliance with an indicator is more useful than learning that 121 of 142 records were in compliance.

By the same reasoning, prepare reports in simple, easy-to-read formats—graphs or control charts are much more meaningful for staff than written reports. Simple checklists like those used to review records also are more useful than running text. Be sure to include brief notes describing identified problems. If you will present the reports to an oversight committee, also include actions already taken by the department.

However the reporting structure is set up for ongoing reviews, make sure you follow up with reports to ensure resolution to all identified noncompliance issues. This information will be helpful at the time of the periodic performance review and at the time of surveys. For example, if your ongoing records review shows that you are in compliance with elements of performance but findings are negative at the time of your on-site survey, the surveyors will be willing to look at your data. This might make or break your survey outcome, or at least give you ammunition when you respond to survey findings. And, of course, with any successful PI project, sustained improvement is the goal. See Chapters 6 and 12 for examples of reporting ongoing records review findings.

Documentation problems that relate to processes

Documentation problems will usually relate to processes rather than to individuals. For example, concurrent record review has identified that, in general, outpatient surgery records do not always have the history and physical reports documented prior to surgery. In addition, the reports that are documented do not include an examination of the heart, lungs, mental status, and body system related to the procedure. Because these problems are process-related, the oversight committee, after review of the graphical report, refers them to the surgery department chair and the Health Information Management director so they can develop a corrective action plan.

Documentation problems that relate to individuals

Although resolution for most records review findings will relate to a process, there may be situations in which an individual physician or hospital employee is identified as the source of a problem. To address such an issue, the committee or team can have direct contact with the person or can refer the findings to the appropriate department director.

Some findings may require action by the medical staff executive committee (or even by the board). If you have identified timely completion of records as a major issue, for example, it may take medical executive committee (MEC) action to impose a stricter policy for records completion.

It will also be the MEC's responsibility to decide whether findings from ongoing reviews, as well as those related to timely completion of records, become part of the physician's credentials file. Because records completion is so important to patient care (and to a successful Joint Commission survey), this information should become a part of the credentials file and be considered at the time of reappointment. Some departments may use individual findings at the time of the annual evaluation. See Chapter 11 for a case study about a hospital that uses its ongoing records review results as part of annual evaluation and its PPR.

Centralize your files

Regardless of who solves the problems, the results should flow back to the facilitator and the oversight group for safekeeping. At the time of the on-site survey, it will be much easier to have documentation of the organization's ongoing records review activities filed in one place. The records will also speak for themselves during the on-site survey. Although surveyors probably will not ask to review documentation of the ongoing records review program if the organization's medical records are in order, it is better to be safe than sorry.

CHAPTER 5

Monitoring timeliness of records completion

Timely and complete documentation

The Joint Commission standards continue to emphasize the timeliness of records completion. In fact, the overview of the *Comprehensive Accreditation Manual for Hospitals'* (CAMH's) Management of Information (IM) chapter states that "ensuring timely and easy access to complete information throughout the organization"[1] is necessary to effectively and continuously improve information management.

As mentioned in Chapter 1, reviewing records for timeliness and completion is part of the ongoing records review process. Element of performance (EP) 8 under IM.6.10 requires the organization to have a policy and procedure on the timely entry of all significant information into patients' medical records. EP 9 also requires the organization to define a complete record and the time frame within which the record must be completed (not to exceed 30 days after discharge). These familiar requirements are no less important in the new accreditation process and, in fact, will be even more important now. See Figure 5.1 for EPs that address timeliness and completion of records.

Other standards, particularly in the "Provision of Care, Treatment, and Services" chapter of the CAMH, continue to specify time requirements for entries such as nursing assessments, history and physical (H&P) reports, and restraints. Although this list does not include all of The Joint Commission standards related to timeliness of medical record entries, it does imply that reviewing timeliness is an important aspect of medical record management. This chapter describes The Joint Commission's emphasis on the completion of records and offers guidance and ideas for tackling this ongoing challenge.

Is timely documentation still a problem?

Medical record completion was a problem well before The Joint Commission existed. In 1919, when the American College of Surgeons first set minimum standards for hospitals, the standards included a mandate for accurate and complete records for all patients—and defined "complete" much as The

CHAPTER FIVE

Figure 5.1

EPs related to timeliness and completion

Standard IM.6.10
The hospital has a complete and accurate medical record for patients assessed, cared for, treated, or served.

EP 8. The hospital has a policy and procedures on the timely entry of all significant information into the patient's medical record.

EP 9. The organization defines a complete record and time frame within which the record must be completed after discharge, not to exceed 30 days after discharge.

EP 10. The hospital measures medical record delinquency at regular intervals, at least every three months.

EP 11. The medical record delinquency rate averaged from the past four quarterly measurements is not greater than 50% of the average monthly discharge (AMD) rate, and no quarterly measurement is greater than 50% of the AMD rate.

Note: The score for EP 11 will result from the following condition described below.

The medical record delinquency rate averaged from the past four quarterly measurements is the following:

- Not greater than 50% of the AMD rate, and no single quarterly measurement is greater than 50% of the AMD rate. The score will be 2—compliance.
- Not greater than 50% of the AMD rate, but one or more quarterly measurements are greater than 50% of the AMD rate. The score will be 1—partial compliance.
- Greater than 50% of the AMD rate, but less than twice (200%) of the AMD rate. The score will be 0—insufficient compliance.
- Equal to or greater than twice (200%) of the AMD rate. The score will be 0—insufficient compliance and a decision of conditional accreditation.

Note: See www.jointcommission.org for a delinquent record statistical form to be completed at the time of on-site surveys.

Source: www.jointcommission.org; 2006 Comprehensive Accreditation Manual for Hospitals, "Management of Information" chapter, Oakbrook Terrace, IL: The Joint Commission.

Joint Commission does today. By 1929, however, records completion was a known problem: Indeed, the Association of Record Librarians of North America, the precursor to the American Health Information Management Association (AHIMA), devoted part of its first annual meeting to the issue.

Today, hospitals continue to receive low scores related to timely documentation of operative reports, documentation of postoperative progress notes, and delinquent medical records after discharge. Numerous other requirements for timely documentation are also problematic. For example, The Joint Commission frequently cites documentation of time-limited orders for restraints in its hospital surveys.

Why is timely record completion so important?

The Joint Commission is serious about records timeliness and completion. Surveyors frequently cite hospitals for failing to meet basic records completion requirements related to delinquent records.

Surveyors look to medical records documentation in the open records more and more frequently as evidence that the hospital carries out its policies and procedures in many clinical and administrative areas, including patient rights, patient education, leadership, and the medical staff. In addition to the fact that The Joint Commission takes timely documentation seriously, it is critically important to patient care, both during and after treatment.

What's changed?

Nothing much has changed in The Joint Commission standards related to delinquent records.

Even though the delinquent rates continue to be calculated based upon "overall" delinquent rates, it is a good idea to keep track of the types of delinquencies. For example, are most of your records delinquent because reports are not dictated or because documents are unsigned? Because timeliness and completeness are parts of ongoing records review requirements (IM.6.10, EP 11), the organization can use this data to good advantage in helping to identify both targeted document types and departments or individuals for focused reviews.

If it wishes to do so, the organization still can include in its records review calculations any outpatient record that is analyzed in the delinquent records calculations. Some organizations may continue to include other caregivers besides physicians in their incomplete record analysis, although doing so can be very time-consuming and is usually a manual process, as most computer systems do not accommodate other caregivers. Therefore, focus on physician record completion for the incomplete record analysis and delinquent process after discharge. Leave identification of timely completion problems for other disciplines to address as part of their records review process. If you have problems with incomplete or late entries (e.g., by nurses, dietitians, therapists, etc.), a good open records review process will identify such issues quickly.

Administrative support

At the heart of timely records completion is a straightforward medical staff policy that is enforced fairly and without exception. The problem with an unclear policy is that it allows physicians to interpret it however they please. However, even the clearest policy set by well-meaning medical staff will be undermined if no one enforces it or if it allows for exceptions. Thus, along with the policy, hospital administration and medical staff leaders must have the fortitude to defend the policy to medical staff members and enforce it even when such enforcement is unpleasant.

HIM department support

For records completion activities to be successful, the records-processing cycle (i.e., the time from patient discharge through records completion) must be as short as possible. This ensures that incomplete records are available for physicians to complete for as long as possible. Some organizations use the date of availability as their starting point to measure how long it takes to complete records. Because regulatory agencies and The Joint Commission use date of discharge, however, facilities should use the discharge date and revamp their records-analysis process to support it.

The delay in getting the records of discharged patients to physicians for completion often stems from the difficulty of retrieving applicable records from nursing units. Hospitals have instituted various methods of quickly collecting discharged patients' records, including having health information management (HIM) staff make rounds several times a day to pick up records on units. Some HIM departments have added records-analysis staff to evening shifts to help make records available to physicians the day after patients are discharged. Other departments have set up a concurrent process to analyze the record by the time of discharge.

Even if technology, such as document imaging and electronic signature, is available in the organization, good ways to track completion of medical records must continue to be part of the process. Availability of technology will speed up records completion and allow for timely authentication at the point of care. When physicians have electronic access to their medical records via the computer, they tend to improve the timeliness of their documentation. Here are some words of advice for those organizations that are planning to set up electronic access for records completion, however: Don't give physicians a choice. Once you establish electronic charting, document imaging, and electronic signature, everyone must participate. Make it clear that the paper record is going away.

Most HIM departments have computerized systems that allow staff to enter missing information into each record and to track the number and status of incomplete records. As stated in previous chapters, such systems also allow the HIM manager to present regular statistics to an oversight committee assigned to track compliance with record requirements.

Physician motivation and support

Although it is in physicians' best interests to complete records quickly and fully, records completion, if not electronic, can still be a paperwork chore that takes busy doctors away from their patients. Therefore, make the process as easy as possible for doctors. Set up a process for timely charting of transcribed reports and easy access to medical records, regardless of whether the access is electronic or in the HIM department.

Some hospitals use disincentives to motivate physicians, such as limiting admission or surgical privileges of physicians with delinquent records. Others use a more positive approach by offering incentives such as food, assistance, and friendly reminders. Figure 5.2 presents 64 ideas that hospitals use to cajole physicians into completing records.

Perhaps the strongest support you can have in this effort is a physician champion. This person may be the chair of the medical record committee, the chair of the performance improvement committee, or the chair of the medical executive committee. He or she should be someone who completes records on time and who has the respect of the entire medical staff. A physician champion who sets a good example and is not afraid to take a stand and to confront his or her peers can go a long way toward solving the delinquent record dilemma.

CHAPTER FIVE

Figure 5.2

64 tips for improving timeliness of records completion

Management support

1. As part of the medical records-tracking system, produce regular reports showing the number of days after discharge that records are completed.

2. Keep basic records completion data in a database. Present that information to the committee/team in charge of medical records timeliness so it has an ongoing look at completion cycles. Implement a computerized tracking system.

3. Present such information graphically. It's generally more meaningful to the committee in that form.

4. Compare delinquency percentages to patient volume so offenders stand out.

5. Provide pleasant, clean, and neat areas in which physicians can complete records. Paint. Try not to have stacks of records lying around.

6. Send records needing to be signed to physicians via courier service or fax. If physicians don't sign the reports in two days, discontinue the service.

7. Use physician extenders to dictate history and physicals, with the attending physician countersigning them within 24 hours.

8. If physicians don't complete their discharge summaries on time, have a resident complete the documentation and send the physician a bill for the time.

9. Find out what physicians prefer—the specific days and times most convenient to them for record completion. Then tell each physician that the department can have the incomplete records ready at his or her preferred time. All physicians are not equal—determine what works for each one and use it.

10. Ask physicians to call the health information management (HIM) department a few minutes or hours before they plan to complete records. That way, staff can have records ready for the physician.

Figure 5.2 (cont.)

64 tips for improving timeliness of records completion

11. Establish a rule that all incomplete records must remain in the department (with the exception of those for patient care). If incomplete records are needed for other reasons, such as quality review, staff must come to the department to review them.

12. During concurrent review, before flagging a record for a missing report, check the dictation system to determine whether it's been dictated.

13. Assign different colored stickers to each physician. Then, as staff review records for completion, they signal missing items by the color unique to the physician responsible.

14. Use color-coding—red is especially noticeable—to indicate documents that need immediate signing, such as operative reports.

15. On admission, put a records completion checklist on the front of the chart and have everyone who puts any documentation in the record indicate when that's accomplished. Doing so eliminates work for the HIM department after the patient is discharged and makes missing elements obvious to the attending physician.

16. Make sure that every physician has equal access to records after discharge. The system of putting records in one physician's file until he or she completes them, then moving them to the next physician's file, and the next, simply doesn't work. It's better to file records by terminal digit or in numerical order so that all physicians have equal access.

17. Go to the nursing unit to retrieve records of discharged patients when necessary.

18. Create satellite areas on nursing units where records staff consolidate incomplete records.

19. Rotate staff who perform deficiency analysis with those who help the physicians with record completion. Doing so gives both groups a better appreciation of the physicians' problems.

20. Have unit staff assemble the record as much as possible at patient discharge. The HIM staff can simply add transcribed or late documents, thus more quickly getting records to the physician for completion. Better yet, institute a "universal" chart order, and don't reassemble after discharge.

Figure 5.2 (cont.)

64 tips for improving timeliness of records completion

21. Have evening clerks on the units or in the HIM department assemble, analyze, and file the day's discharges so the records are ready for physicians the next morning.

22. Make sure someone who is cross-trained in record completion policies is available to physicians at all times.

Administrative support

23. Make sure records completion statistics are part of the consideration for recredentialing each physician.

24. Create and enforce a time frame shorter than 30 days for record completion. A requirement of 15 days, for example, gives 15 extra days for the hospital to make sure that all items are completed.

25. It's basic, but hospital administration as well as medical staff leaders must uphold the requirements for medical record completion. And these requirements must apply to every physician, because making exceptions sends the message that the hospital is not serious about the matter.

26. Make sure the president of the medical staff, or another person whom physicians respect, stresses—at every opportunity—the value of timely records completion, what is required of physicians for records completion, and the process for completion.

27. Reduce the number of unsigned verbal orders by restricting them to emergencies only. Define "emergency."

28. Work with other hospitals in the system or in the city to make records completion requirements—including disincentives—consistent across all hospitals. That way physicians cannot use the threat of taking their business elsewhere.

29. Have the HIM department call any physicians with delinquent records.

30. Add a part-time position of physician liaison to the staff, and make follow-up on delinquent records his or her responsibility.

Figure 5.2 (cont.)

64 tips for improving timeliness of records completion

31. Have the vice president of medical affairs call the department chairs of delinquent surgeons to tell them to cancel their surgeries until records are complete.

32. Don't allow delinquent physicians to preregister patients for admissions or schedule surgeries. Apply the policy to both inpatients and outpatients.

Physician motivation

33. Hold "dine and sign" lunches.

34. Make speakerphones available to physicians dictating in the HIM department. When using them, physicians have their hands free to shuffle pages in the medical records.

35. Help physicians make the most of their time in the HIM department by separating the records that need signing from the ones that need dictation.

36. Notify the medical executive committee about any physicians who are on the suspension list for three consecutive incomplete records. Require the physician to come before the executive committee to explain his or her reasons for delinquent records. Put a copy in the credentials file.

37. Keep several hand-held dictation units available for physicians to borrow for dictation in their cars or when they are away from a phone.

38. Help surgeons and anesthesiologists by taking all their incomplete records to the physicians' area in the recovery room. Even better, monitor the surgery schedules, and if a physician with incomplete records is scheduled to do surgery, take his or her records to the operating room lounge.

39. Establish a "mini" chart room in the obstetrical lounge so the obstetricians can complete records while waiting for mothers to deliver.

40. Take incomplete records to physicians when they gather for medical staff committee, continuing education, and staff meetings.

Chapter Five

Figure 5.2 (cont.)

64 tips for improving timeliness of records completion

41. Take records to the physicians' lounge or surgery records to the surgery lounge for completion between operations.

42. Use food as an enticement. Managers use all sorts of goodies to encourage physicians to come to the HIM department—from cookies, candy, popcorn, and coffee to continental breakfasts and even weekly lunches.

43. Remember that some physicians are colorblind; for those physicians, use striped tags to ensure they can readily locate their required documentation.

44. Identify medical staff members who miss signing documents and offer to have staff review their records as they are being completed.

45. Hold a contest for residents to see who dictates the most discharge summaries on the day of discharge.

46. Rather than suspending the admitting privileges for one physician, suspend them for the physician's entire group.

47. If there are several hospitals in a system, suspend the physician at all of the hospitals.

48. Keep up with record delinquencies by clinical department and increase or decrease the budget yearly based on record performance.

49. Publicize, through bulletin boards or medical staff newsletters, the names of physicians who complete their records on time or the names of the worst offenders.

50. Fine residents who fail to complete records on time or withhold their paychecks until they complete records. Tougher still: Make each resident complete all of his or her records before allowing him or her to graduate.

51. Use physician pressure on residents. Assign the job of policing medical records completion to the chief of service rather than to residents. Or suspend the admitting physician along with the resident when a record is delinquent. Or institute a policy that if the resident has

Figure 5.2 (cont.)

64 tips for improving timeliness of records completion

not signed a record within so many days, the record becomes the responsibility of the attending physician.

52. Suspend other needed services when physicians have delinquent records, such as providing copies of dictated reports that physicians need for billing.

53. Give physicians who have incomplete records personal treatment by calling their offices to alert them and by offering staff help as they complete records.

54. Many disincentives and incentives work, but a survey that **Medical Records Briefing**, an HCPro newsletter, conducted several years ago showed that rapport with physicians was second only to suspension of privileges in its effectiveness.

55. Use interdepartmental mail or couriers to hand-deliver notices of incomplete records or delinquent records.

56. Put notices of incomplete or delinquent records on brightly colored stationery and envelopes so they stand out from the physicians' regular mail.

57. When the physician signs on to any hospital computer, program the screen to flash if any records are incomplete. Or give a list of physicians with delinquent records to the front office of the hospital and ask staff to notify the HIM department when these physicians come in.

58. Use humor. A cartoon or poem sent with the notices of incomplete or delinquent records may get attention when a severe warning does not.

59. After records are incomplete for several days, send a reminder to the physicians every week. And send a weekly list of physicians with delinquent records to their department chairs.

60. Use quality improvement tools to determine why records aren't complete. Don't assume that records are incomplete simply because physicians hate to do them. Instead, look more deeply at the problem to determine whether forms need redesigning, physicians need reeducating, or equipment causes more obstacles than it corrects. Make sure the HIM department's processes are efficient and timely.

Figure 5.2 (cont.)

64 tips for improving timeliness of records completion

61. Many hospitals find that the number of forms has grown out of control. A review of the forms in use will likely find many that are unwieldy, redundant, or confusing. Fewer, better-designed forms may facilitate record completion. Ask for physician input in the process of reviewing, reducing, and redesigning forms.

62. Use electronic signature software for signing reports.

63. Reduce the number of items you require for record completion, if state and federal laws allow.

64. Implement electronic records that provide access to physicians from any location, inside and outside the organization, for viewing and completing medical records.

Electronic health records support

Many of these tips have proven successful; however, they also tend to put the burden on the HIM department, which must get the physicians to do a better job at documentation and records completion.

Therefore, the best solution in this day and age of electronic health records is to use technology to improve documentation, ensure timely completion of records, and assist with holding physicians and other caregivers responsible for their documentation. Voice recognition dictation, electronic signature, computerized physician order entry, and other electronic medical record (EMR) solutions to improve nursing staff, emergency department, and operating room documentation are the answers to improving documentation and timely completion of medical records.

If you don't have an EMR but are considering one, use a Request for Proposal process. This is a process whereby vendors come in to demonstrate their products at your hospital, which gives all your staff a chance to see and discuss the products. Because legible, accurate, and complete medical records are the goal of every HIM department, consider products that computerize physician and nursing documentation first. Products that include document imaging (which allow staff to scan paper forms and records into the medical record) are also a big plus.

Choosing the right vendor is a major decision for your hospital. HIM plays a vital role in the decision, but other parties that must be involved in the selection process include the information technology department, nursing leadership, representatives from clinical departments (e.g., laboratory, radiology), and physicians. Include people who will actually be using the product.

Even though EMR and scanning systems cost a lot of money, in the long run they will pay for themselves in time, staffing, and improved patient care.

Endnote

1. Joint Commission on Accreditation of Healthcare Organizations, 2007 *Comprehensive Accreditation Manual for Hospitals*, "Management of Information" chapter, Oakbrook Terrace, IL: The Joint Commission.

CHAPTER 6

Demonstrating compliance to The Joint Commission surveyors

Introduction

Although The Joint Commission has eliminated the closed medical record review session, it is still a good idea to have documented proof of your ongoing records review process. As stated earlier, if findings during survey indicate noncompliance for timely history and physical (H&P) reports, having such proof would allow you to show surveyors that ongoing reviews indicate a different story. It is also important to validate compliance when completing the annual periodic performance review. A well-planned program will ensure continuous compliance.

Ongoing record review policies, procedures, and written plans

Every organization should ensure that its policies and procedures cover the functions of its ongoing medical records review program. Policies should state the responsibilities of medical staff physicians as well as the authority of the review committee, departments, or team(s). The policies and procedures should clearly indicate the time limits for records completion so physicians are fully aware of how quickly they must complete their medical records. Generally, time limits for records completion are found in the medical staff rules and regulations. Examples of how you might word this appear in Figures 6.1 and 6.2.

Organizations should draft written plans that contain the following sections for ongoing records review programs (also see Figure 2.2 for a medical records committee protocol):

- **Purpose:** A brief, written statement that the organization is committed to assessing medical record documentation.

Figure 6.1

A complete record

Medical record entries are to be made in a timely manner, and the record is complete when

- its content reflects the patient's condition on arrival, diagnosis, test results, therapy, condition and in-hospital progress, and condition at discharge

- its contents, including any required clinical resume or final progress notes, are assembled and authenticated as required

- all final diagnoses and complications are recorded without the use of symbols or abbreviations

Figure 6.2

Delinquent records

Medical records will be considered delinquent thirty (30) days after discharge. At the time of discharge, records incomplete due to failure to complete and sign the history and physical report, operative report(s), consultation(s), verbal/telephone orders, or discharge summary will be available in the HIM department for physicians to complete.

- **Responsibilities:** A statement identifying the group or groups responsible for ongoing review and the functions for which the group(s) are responsible. For example, this section could state that the health information management (HIM) department collects the data from reviews and that it prepares and distributes reports from them.

- **Scope:** A section stating that ongoing records review includes both inpatients and outpatients and all services provided.

- **Topics:** A section outlining how to select topics and any specific ongoing topics. You could base topics upon types of documents, documenters, or clinical service groups. For example, H&Ps

and operative reports; pain management; diagnoses; nurses, doctors, physical therapists; or cardiology, surgery, and obstetrics, to name a few.

- **Indicators:** If indicators for the items under review are available, include them in the plan. At a minimum, the plan should state that the organization will use the indicators addressed in IM.6.10, element of performance (EP) 11, as appropriate to the topics under review. In most cases, organizations should expect 100% compliance with the EPs. Compliance requirements should dictate how you determine when the findings from ongoing record reviews warrant focused studies.

- **Process:** A section describing how data is collected and reported.

- **Action and reporting:** A statement identifying the committees, departments, or teams that will take action in response to problems identified through ongoing records review, what actions they may take, and to whom they report.

- **Statement of confidentiality:** A statement that all those participating in ongoing records review honor patients' rights to privacy, protect medical information, and report only information that is stripped of patient identifiers.

Note: Organizations may modify or add to the above sections when drafting their plans. They also may refer to the above sections by different names.

Forms, minutes, and reports

In addition to its policies, procedures, and plan, the organization should assemble documentation that shows that the program actually works. As stated before, use easy-to-read, graphical formats to illustrate the results of reviews and actions taken to improve processes.

For example, organizations should continue to assemble the minutes of involved committees and teams, which reflect ongoing review activities and actions taken to resolve problems. They also should report ongoing records review activities to appropriate leadership. Figures 6.3 and 6.4 are examples that you can use to report ongoing review activities to the oversight group and the appropriate leadership.

Chapter Six

Compile the report in Microsoft Word or Excel. Graphs, pie charts, or other types of visual displays can accompany the report. Attach an action plan to any indicator that has been noncompliant for two reporting periods. Organizations may choose to continue using the summary report that The Joint Commission required prior to 2004, although it is no longer required—it is nonetheless an example of one way to report the ongoing activities of records review. Chapter 11 provides other examples of such reports.

Figure 6.3

Ongoing records review report

Compliant		Noncompliant	
Department: Surgery department			
Indicator	**Target**	**YTD actual**	
1. H&P on chart prior to surgery	100%	95%	
2. Postoperative progress note written immediately after surgery	100%	100%	
Actions taken to address noncompliant indicators:			

Figure 6.4

Quarterly summary report

Ongoing records review

	Q-1	Q-2	Q-3	Q-4
# of open records reviewed	(M/NM)			
Indicators				
1.				
2.				
3.				
Focus reviews				
1.				
2.				
3.				
Patient tracer reviews				
1.				
2.				
3.				
Other reviews				
1.				
2.				
3.				
# of closed records reviewed				
1.				
2.				
3.				
Delinquent records stats				

Comments:

Actions taken:

M = met; NM = not met

CHAPTER 7

Incorporating the tracer methodology into ongoing records review

Accurate, complete, legible, and timely medical records will continue to be essential elements for periodic performance reviews and on-site surveys, particularly as The Joint Commission rolls out its new tracer methodology during surveys.

How tracers work

Tracer methodology uses actual patients to assess how hospitals care for patients and comply with relevant standards. Medical records play an important role in this new process. Surveyors will randomly select patients—and subsequently, their medical records—at the beginning of the survey. The surveyors will visit the units, sites, or departments in the exact sequence, when possible, experienced by the patients selected.

For example, a patient is admitted through the emergency department (ED) and admitted to the cardiology unit, where he has a cardiac catheterization. He receives x-rays, lab work, and medications; is put on a special diet; and is transferred to the cardiac rehabilitation unit after discharge. The surveyor would follow—or trace—the patient's path and talk to the direct caregivers who provided care and treatment to the patient. Thus, The Joint Commission has given this process the name "tracer."

Surveyors will generally select open records for this review; however, it's possible for a surveyor to request closed records if a patient was a recent readmission. Other closed records requests could result from the inability to locate enough patients hospitalized at the time of survey—if surveyors wish to trace patients in restraints, for example, and none are available. Open or closed, quality medical records have never been more important.

The Joint Commission can better assess compliance with standards related to operational systems and processes based upon the actual experience of the patient. Surveyors do so by looking at the entire sequence of care provided to the patient rather than reviewing a few records in each department against a checklist, as was the format in previous surveys.

CHAPTER SEVEN

How documentation fits in

Because The Joint Commission uses the medical record as the road map to identify what treatments the patient received and who the caregivers were, documentation must be as timely and complete as possible. The medical record should accurately reflect the patient's care and treatment from start to finish. Late or illegible entries and otherwise poor documentation do not contribute to the quality and safety of patient care and will not contribute to a successful survey under the new process.

Joint Commission surveyors perform system tracers, such as medication management, information/data flow, and infection control, at the time of survey, and use the medical record to assess the effectiveness of the processes and systems the hospital has in place. For example, the attending physician places a telephone order for medication to the ED when her patient presents for treatment. The medication is given without review by the pharmacist or the ED doctor. The patient has an adverse reaction, and it is not properly reported. When the surveyor reviews the medical record, the documentation reveals that the telephone order was not verified and the patient received the wrong medication. The record documents the medication reaction, but when the surveyor talks to the caregiver, it is revealed that the reaction was not reported according to policy. In this scenario, there is definitely a problem with the management of medication, and the review of the record has validated a broken process identified in a system tracer.

This example also illustrates how important it is for organizations to conduct mock patient and system tracers. If it had done so, the organization in the example would have found the problem before the surveyor did. It also would have familiarized staff with the new methodology, helped improve documentation, trained staff to speak up, identified opportunities for improvement, and helped develop well-functioning clinical and treatment teams.

How to work tracer methodology into ongoing records review

But how do you use tracers for ongoing records review? This book outlines traditional methods for review, which are still useful and should be included in your ongoing review processes, but using the tracer methodology as part of your regular ongoing records review will prove valuable as well. It will alert reviewers to the importance of timely and accurate documentation in the medical record and will help your staff know what to expect during the actual survey. More important, it will help to identify inconsistencies in care and documentation, as well as demonstrate the importance of communication and teamwork among caregivers.

Identify PFAs and CSGs

To get started in using tracers as part of your ongoing records review, first put yourself in the place of the surveyors. What will they do? They will know the standards and elements of performance (EPs), the National Patient Safety Goals (NPSGs), the organization's priority focus areas (PFAs), and clinical service groups (CSGs). (Note: You should be able to access your own PFAs and CSGs on your organization's secured Joint Commission Web site, The Joint Commission Connect™).

Examples of PFAs are assessment and care, communication, information management, and infection control. CSGs include cardiac surgery, oncology, orthopedics, and psychiatry, to name a few. Both are based upon the organization's specific data and services that it provides, and this information helps surveyors determine which patients they should trace. Therefore, your first steps toward incorporating tracers into ongoing records review will be to

- identify
    - the organization's CSGs
    - the organization's PFAs
    - the patients
- select the CSGs and PFAs that will be the focus of the reviews

As mentioned in previous chapters, the organization can determine who will participate in ongoing records review. However, when using the tracer methodology for reviews, it becomes even more important to use currently active patients in the hospital for your reviews and caregivers as your reviewers. The health information management (HIM) staff, as usual, can help facilitate the process.

Decide how to conduct the review

Try conducting the reviews either at the department level, which helps get the appropriate staff involved, or through a team approach of reviewing recently discharged records. One hospital started its tracer approach to ongoing reviews by introducing the concept during the monthly nursing team leader meeting. The HIM director brought recently discharged records to the monthly meetings and asked teams of two nurses to review one record. After the reviews were completed, the teams presented their findings. It was an eye-opener for the reviewers, who have replicated the process on their units.

Chapter Seven

Basically, getting started requires the following steps:

1. Identify the reviewers
2. Identify the process (at the units or after discharge)
3. Select the records
4. Review the records and chart the path of the patient
5. Review the records and record issues related to documentation

There are numerous benefits to using this methodology for chart reviews, but the primary one is that the process immediately identifies issues and validates the importance of accurate and timely medical records.

Tips for taking a tracer approach to records review

Because the requirements for ongoing records review are basically left up to the organization, this approach can work when others have failed. Here are a few tips to consider if you decide to take the tracer approach to records reviews:

1. **Focus on the quality of documentation. Here are some sample questions to ask:**
   - Does the record clearly reflect that the care and treatment provided to the patient are appropriate and given in the most beneficial and necessary time? For example, are the assessments and treatments for pain meaningful to the patient's condition?

   - Is the plan of care based upon documented communication between the physician and the other caregivers, or does it look fragmented? Is it truly interdisciplinary?

   - Does the treatment appear to be appropriate for the diagnosis?

2. *Focus on timely entries. Examine the following entries for timely documentation as you conduct a tracer review:*
   - History and physicals (H&Ps)
   - Nursing assessments
   - Response to referrals
   - Informed consents
   - Operative reports

3. *Focus on legibility. Are all entries legible and free from abbreviations not approved for use?*

Summary

The bottom line is that the record should reflect that care is consistent with policies and procedures, that the appropriate coordination and communication takes place among the healthcare team members caring for the patient (e.g., staff, departments, and physicians), and that handoffs of information occur appropriately and in a timely manner.

Figure 7.1 provides an example of a tracer case study that illustrates documentation issues. Figure 7.2 is a tool to use when conducting a patient tracer to identify documentation issues. Figure 7.3 is another example of a tool that you could use for chart reviews during tracers. Figure 7.4 offers an example of a tool you can use when conducting a system tracer for information management.

Using patient and system tracers for ongoing records review will take the mundane out of the process, teach staff what to expect at the time of survey, and improve your medical records—all at the same time.

Use a generic tracer tool to train other departments

When all is said and done, the use of a generic patient tracer tool that covers requirements for all departments, as well as ongoing record review items, is the best method to ensure compliance and readiness for an unannounced survey. Nursing units and other departments can use this tool to determine their own compliance and readiness for a survey by conducting internal tracers, focusing on

Chapter Seven

their department instead of chasing a patient around a hospital (like a true tracer review). Figure 7.5 provides an example of a comprehensive tracer tool.

Another good strategy for departmental training is to create a "tracer team." This team conducts tracers on a regular basis by following patients throughout the organization, much like The Joint Commission surveyors will do at the time of a real unannounced survey. And like real unannounced surveys, the tracer team should not let departments know in advance that it is coming.

For example, if you conduct a mock tracer review of your radiology department, here's a typical process to consider:

- Talk to the radiology techs. Go through the National Patient Safety Goals—ask whether they use two patient identifiers, for example.
- Look in the medical record for documentation of invasive procedures. Make sure there is documentation of consent, an H&P, etc.
- Conduct environment rounding to make sure staff have tested their equipment and fire extinguishers on a monthly basis, have clean refrigerators, and keep a refrigerator log.
- Check for proper security of medications and contrast media.
- Determine whether pharmacists are reviewing orders for medications.
- If your hospital uses an electronic health records system, have a staff member operate the computer to make sure he or she is properly entering information into the record and can find the right pieces of information in the patient's chart.

If you use the tracer team approach as part of ongoing record reviews or as a supplement to other reviews, remember to report your findings and establish accountability. Senior leadership from the HIM department is a good candidate for holding these departments accountable. And remember to maintain a regular schedule for tracer team practice runs.

To have success during an actual survey, it's crucial to perform regular tracers. Include leadership as part of the team, include a comprehensive tool, and provide immediate feedback to departmental managers to assure success. It's better to be prepared ahead of time than not be ready when the surveyor visits the department or nursing unit.

Figure 7.1

Tracer case study

Priority focus areas: Assessment, care, communication, staffing, infection control, medication use, information management based upon clinical/ service groups

The patient is a 28-year-old male diabetic who was admitted three days ago because of persistent fever. Several days before admission, he developed low-grade fever, headache, cough, and abdominal pain. Tylenol did not reduce the temperature. Two days prior to admission, his temperature rose to 103°F, and he took acetaminophen and ibuprofen without relief of the fever. Two days before admission (Friday), he came to the emergency room (ER). Physical exam and chest x-ray were normal. A blood specimen and sputum cultures were drawn. The next day (Saturday), the blood culture yielded gram-negative rods, and the sputum culture was negative. The patient was admitted on Sunday. The admission assessment data revealed that the patient appeared tired and thin but not acutely ill. Hematologic tests, blood chemistry, and CT scan with contrast of abdomen and pelvis were performed.

Tracer findings:

ER visit
- Review of medical record did not indicate patient was called back on Saturday about the positive blood culture, nor were the lab results on the medical record.

- ✓ Surveyor began the tracer by visiting the ER. She questioned staff about their policy on calling back patients with positive lab results. Was the policy the same for weekends as weekdays? She asked about the turnaround time for charting lab reports and whether reports were available on the computer.

Inpatient visit
- Review of the medical record showed no evidence that that pain had been assessed.

- There was no documentation regarding allergies.

- Several abbreviations from the prohibited list were found in the medical record.

- Nutritional screening on admission revealed a referral to the clinical dietitian, but no documented evidence that he had visited the patient.

Figure 7.1 (cont.)

Tracer case study

- No history and physical (H&P) on the medical record.

✓ Surveyor asked to speak with nurse in charge of patient. Questioned policy related to pain assessment and how often pain was assessed. Asked for policy related to documenting allergies. Made note to discuss informed consent at time of radiology visit. Made note to review prohibited abbreviations list and check for use in other medical records. Made note to discuss response to referrals when talking with dietitian. Made note to review medical staff rule/regulations related to H&Ps.

Staffing and infection control

- At the time of the inpatient visit, surveyor talked with nurse manager about staffing, control of medications, and handwashing techniques used by staff. Nurse manager stated that unit was staffed with 25% traveling nurses.

✓ Surveyor made note of two travelers for review of their personnel files.

Patient interview

- Patient could not remember if anyone had asked him about an advance directive or his level of pain; was not aware of risk related to contrast media.

✓ Surveyor requested policy for advance directives.

Lab visit

- Determined that lab maintained quality control of glucose-monitoring devices.

Radiology visit

- No informed consent was signed for contrast studies, and the department did not have a process to inform patients about reactions to contrast media.

INCORPORATING THE TRACER METHODOLOGY INTO ONGOING RECORDS REVIEW

Figure 7.2

Patient tracer data collection form

MR#_____   Admit date _____

Clinical service group (CSG): _____
(This is the service the patient was admitted to; for example, OB, cardiac, surgical)

Priority focus areas (PFAs):

Processes, systems, or structures in a healthcare organization that significantly affect the quality and safety of care. For today's chart review, look for supportive documentation in the following PFAs:

1. Assessment (H&P, nursing assessment)
2. Communication (handoffs, verbal/telephone order RB/V, "time out" before procedure, unapproved abbreviations, other issues related to communication)
3. Medication management (legible, signed, appropriate to the patient's condition)
4. Rights and ethics (advance directives, informed consent)
5. Other documentation issues

Path of the patient

1. _____
2. _____
3. _____
4. _____
5. _____

Unit/Dept.	Caregivers	Issues	PFA(s)

ONGOING RECORDS REVIEW, FIFTH EDITION   © 2007 HCPro, Inc.

Chapter Seven

Figure 7.3

Open/active chart review form

This is not inclusive of all elements in a full medical record review, but focuses on high-risk processes.

Note: Entries must be complete, legible, dated, authenticated, and timely.

Key: P= Present   A= Absent   N/A= Not applicable

Chart	1	2	3	4	5	6	7	8	9	10
Demographics										
H&P timely										
Orders										
Verbal/telephone orders										
Consents for treatment										
Consents for blood										
Advance directives										
Progress notes										
Consults										
Nursing notes										
Medication/effects										
Allergies										
Lab values										
Imaging studies										
Surgical/procedure postop note immediately after surgery/procedure										
Licensed Independent practitioners' assessment immediately prior to moderate sedation/anesthesia										
Compliance with do-not-use abbreviations list										
Pain assessment										
Nutritional screen										
Functional screen										
Barriers to learning assessed										
Psychosocial needs assessed										
End-of-life needs										
Reassessment after change in status										
Education provided to patient/family										
Evidence of interdisciplinary care planning										

Source: Tracer Methodology: Frontline Strategies to Prepare your Organization for JCAHO Survey. Copyright 2004, HCPro, Inc. Reprinted with permission.

Figure 7.4

Priority focus audit form: Information management tracer

Tracer patient: _____

Information management Chart audit, interview with staff, competencies, and observation	Met/2	Partial/1	Not met/0	N/A	Comments
Confidentiality and security of medical record maintained					
Medical record is complete and accurate; contains patient-specific information as appropriate for care, treatment, and services					
Abbreviations, acronyms, and symbols used are standardized					
Do-not-use abbreviation list is evident and meets compliance requirements					
Evidence of process for verbal/telephone order readback					
Data and information is timely					
Current knowledge-based information is readily available to staff and practitioners (including after hours)					
Medical record entries are dated and authenticated according to law and regulation					
Discharge summary present when applicable and contains: Reason for hospitalization Significant findings Procedures/services provided Patient's condition upon discharge Instructions to patient & family					
Closed medical record completed within 30 days					
Medical record delinquency rate below 50%					
Allergies to foods and medications documented in medical record					
List of all medications evident					
H&P within 24 hours					
Current H&P prior to operative procedures					

CHAPTER SEVEN

Figure 7.4 (cont.)

Priority focus audit form: Information management tracer

Information management	Met/2	Partial/1	Not met/0	N/A	Comments
Operative note entered immediately after surgery and contains the following:					
Primary surgeon's name					
Assistant's name					
Findings					
Description of procedure performed					
Estimated blood loss					
Specimens removed					
Postoperative diagnosis					
Assessment by LIP immediately prior to moderate or deep sedation					
For ambulatory patients, a list is generated by the third visit and maintained thereafter with the following information:					
Diagnoses					
Operative/invasive procedures					
Allergies					
Medications (including over-the-counter drugs and herbal preparations)					
Continuity of care is evident in medical record					
Care and treatment is justified in documentation					
Progress notes authenticated and dated					
Orders authenticated and dated					
Orders for restraints per law/regulation					
Restraint monitoring logs evident and complete					
Informed consents signed					
Advance directives indicated, copy on medical record?					
Identification data sheet evident in medical record					
Blood slips complete					
Laboratory data timely					

Source: Tracer Methodology: Frontline Strategies to Prepare your Organization for JCAHO Survey. Copyright 2004, HCPro, Inc. Reprinted with permission.

INCORPORATING THE TRACER METHODOLOGY INTO ONGOING RECORDS REVIEW

Figure 7.5

Patient tracer worksheet

Reviewer's name: _____ Date: _____ Unit: _____

Hospital: _____

Pt name: _____

MR#: _____

Age: _____

Admission date: _____

Anticipated discharge date: _____

Diagnosis: _____

Sequence of care/services:
_____
_____
_____

Staff/Physicians:
_____
_____
_____

Priority focus areas (PFAs):
1. Assessment of care/service
2. Communication
3. Credentialed and privileged practitioners
4. Equipment use
5. Infection control
6. Physical environment
7. Information management
8. Medication management
9. Organizational structure
10. Orientation and training
11. Patient safety/NPSGs
12. Quality improvement
13. Rights and ethics
14. Staffing

PFAs/Questions

Assessment of care/service

☐ Initial nursing assessment completed within eight hours of admission?
☐ H&P within 24 hours of admission AND before surgery?
☐ H&P reviewed/updated if it exceeds 30-day time frame?
☐ Allergies to foods and meds?
☐ Pain assessment on admission, every shift and one hour after intervention; pain scales available and documented?
☐ Nutritional assessment (referrals completed within 48 hours of notification)?

Issues identified/notes

ONGOING RECORDS REVIEW, FIFTH EDITION © 2007 HCPro, Inc. 67

Chapter Seven

Figure 7.5 (cont.)

Patient tracer worksheet

PFAs/Questions	Issues identified/notes
☐ Functional assessment physical therapy referrals completed within 24 hours, and occupational therapy within 48 hours?	
☐ Falls assessment with initial nursing assessment? Patient is reassessed when nursing reassessment is done (when patient status indicates, every 24 hours, or upon transfer to another unit or caregiver)?	
☐ Interdisciplinary plan of care (IPOC) with individual patient goals/needs completed within eight hours?	
☐ Reassessments and updates of IPOC (as needed, every 24 hours, or upon transfer to another unit)?	
☐ Social assessment including language barriers? Appropriate interpretive services provided?	
☐ Patient/family education needs assessed?	
☐ End-of-life care needs assessed—need for advance directives on chart?	
☐ Evidence of plan for discharge/transfer within 72 hours of referral?	
☐ Preanesthesia or premoderate sedation assessment? Patient evaluated again immediately prior to induction?	
☐ Assessment of pain? Reassessment as needed and after pain meds (15–30-minute IV or one-hour oral?)	
☐ Same level of care provided if patient is admitted but still in ED?	
Communication/Documentation	
☐ Medical record entries are signed and dated?	
☐ Strike-outs with one line, initial, and date?	
☐ Verbal orders signed within 48 hours—24 hours for restraints?	
☐ "Time out" for surgery and invasive procedures?	

Figure 7.5 (cont.)

Patient tracer worksheet

PFAs/Questions	Issues identified/notes
☐ "Readback" of verbal orders (write down and read back, and document "RB/V")? ☐ Nurse "readback" of critical test results (write down and read back) and communication to MD/designee within two hours? ☐ Restraints (order for each calendar day in restraint; reason documented; alternatives considered; monitoring every two hours appropriately documented; verbal orders received only by RN—no PRN)? ☐ IPOC documented with care provided by all disciplines? ☐ Patient and family education provided—documented in chart? ☐ Operative note done immediately following surgery? ☐ Patient handoffs documented? Shift change, transfers?	
Credentialed and privileged practitioners ☐ How does staff know if a physician has privileges? ☐ How does staff know whether a physician is credentialed for a specific procedure?	
Equipment use ☐ Clinical alarms audible—how were they tested (maintained on a schedule, tested for audibility)? ☐ Check equipment for preventive maintenance; provide equipment # if overdue. ☐ Check crash carts for daily checks. ☐ Check refrigerator logs and refrigerators to see whether open bottles of meds have been dated.	

Chapter Seven

Figure 7.5 (cont.)

Patient tracer worksheet

PFAs/Questions	Issues identified/notes
Infection control ☐ Tell me how you comply with the Centers for Disease Control and Prevention's hand-hygiene guidelines. ☐ Do you know your department's hand hygiene compliance rate? ☐ Observe staff and MDs washing hands/using alcohol-based hand foam. ☐ Are isolation precautions followed in all areas, including OR, Endoscopy, ED (staff and family)? ☐ Test for negative pressure? ☐ Clean linen covered, bottom enclosed? ☐ Clean room—CLEAN ONLY? ☐ Dirty room neat and clean—nothing on floor? ☐ How do you know whether equipment is clean? ☐ Needle boxes secured—none overfilled? ☐ Storage under sinks (no patient use items that will be damaged by water; no food?)	
Physical environment ☐ No smoking policy—are patients allowed to smoke? ☐ Call buttons within reach? ☐ Bed alarms working? ☐ O2 tanks properly secured? ☐ Doors not propped open? ☐ Appropriate storage and security of meds, including IV fluids? ☐ Temperature logs within acceptable range? ☐ Fire exits free from obstruction?	

Figure 7.5 (cont.)

Patient tracer worksheet

PFAs/Questions	Issues identified/notes
☐ Evacuation plan posted? ☐ Exit signs lighted? ☐ Red fire cards at telephones? ☐ Sprinkler heads unobstructed within 18 inches? ☐ Electrical panels free from obstruction within 3 feet, labeled? ☐ How is oxygen shut off in case of fire? Who does it?	
Information management ☐ No prohibited abbreviations? ☐ Check for legibility/readability in records. ☐ Medical records secure from unauthorized access, computer screens secure? ☐ No computer passwords visible? ☐ Privacy and confidentiality of patient info? ☐ Timeliness of transcription? ☐ Consents, education, other forms appropriate for age group?	
Medication management ☐ Medication carts locked—no drink cups or food? ☐ Secure and safe storage of meds and supplies? ☐ PRN meds need indication or symptom for med, dose, frequency? ☐ Range orders (dose, interval) follow policy? ☐ Multidose vials with 28-day expiration? ☐ Controls for look-alike/sound-alike meds—safety procedures followed? What are they?	

CHAPTER SEVEN

Figure 7.5 (cont.)

Patient tracer worksheet

PFAs/Questions	Issues identified/notes
☐ Medication refrigerator temp logs? ☐ High-risk medications identified and highlighted to staff? Safety procedures followed? ☐ Pharmacy review prior to administration of contrast media? ☐ Diagnosis or indication recorded in medical record for each medication ordered?	
Organizational structure ☐ How are policies communicated? ☐ How do we promote a safe organization for patients? ☐ One standard of care throughout organization? ☐ How are performance improvement strategies and results communicated through channels?	
Orientation and training ☐ Personnel records are current and available: • Job description • Licensure/registration/certification • Orientation: department and organization • Competency: initial and ongoing • Training/education in patient safety, error reporting, and team training • Performance evaluation ☐ Staff training for equipment use ☐ Training and continuing education	

Figure 7.5 (cont.)

Patient tracer worksheet

PFAs/Questions	Issues identified/notes
☐ Competencies and training address age-specific categories: peds, adolescent, adult, geriatric? ☐ Waived testing (blood glucose, urine, H. pylori)? ☐ Are contracted employees (e.g., security) trained?	
Patient safety/NPSGs ☐ Two patient identifiers used and checked against a source document? ☐ "Time out" immediately prior to confirm correct patient, procedure, site, side (including non-OR areas) must be documented. ☐ Preprocedure: Site and procedure verified with schedule and MD order, consent and patient? ☐ Surgical site marked (person doing procedure will initial, patient is involved in process, and it's done prior to moving patient to procedural area)? ☐ "Read back" of verbal/telephone orders and critical test results? ☐ No prohibited abbreviations; what should you do with an order that includes an unapproved abbreviation? (Do not execute until verified and rewritten correctly.) ☐ Hand-hygiene policy followed? ☐ Controls for look-alike/sound-alike medications (including sample meds)? ☐ Medication reconciliation: Are meds reviewed and updated as necessary (including admission, postop, transfer, discharge)? ☐ Patient assessed and reassessed for risk of falling—required actions taken? ☐ Do we have a culture of patient safety?	

Figure 7.5 (cont.)

Patient tracer worksheet

PFAs/Questions	Issues identified/notes
☐ Same-name alerts? ☐ Are patients and family involved in care decisions? ☐ Do you assess patients for potential suicide?	
Quality improvement ☐ Approach to performance improvement (PI)? ☐ Describe any PI activities on unit, changes, data displayed. ☐ Staff knowledge of core measures, if applicable (heart failure, OB, pneumonia)? ☐ Staff knowledge of patient/employee satisfaction scores? ☐ Staff knowledge of definition and procedures for sentinel event/near-miss, including those related to nosocomial infection? ☐ Any applicable sentinel event alerts and responses? ☐ Staff knowledge of last failure modes effects analysis—purpose, impact, methodology? ☐ What is a problem a staff member would most like to see improved?	

Source: Roper St. Francis Healthcare, Charlestown, SC. Reprinted with permission.

Chapter 8

Scoring and decision rules

The Joint Commission changed its scoring guidelines in 2004. The changes make it easier for hospitals to score themselves both on an ongoing basis and at the time of the periodic performance review.

Scoring for standards

Elements of performance (EPs) for each standard are scored as follows:

- 2: Satisfactory compliance
- 1: Partial compliance
- 0: Insufficient compliance
- N/A: Not applicable

Track records and scoring guidelines

Track records (how long you've had a policy or practice in place) are still required and are important criteria for scoring standards. During the triennial survey, surveyors will score based upon the following track records:

- 0 for fewer than six months
- 1 for six to 11 months
- 2 for 12 consecutive months or more

During the **initial survey**, The Joint Commission will score standards based on track records in the following manner:

- 0 for fewer than two months
- 1 for two to three months
- 2 for four months or more

CHAPTER EIGHT

Scoring for elements of performance

Scoring guidelines also involve the specific requirements or EPs listed under each standard. The Joint Commission will score each EP based on three categories: A, B, and C. Each EP is assigned a category, which you can find to the right of each EP in the *Comprehensive Accreditation Manual for Hospitals* (CAMH). It might be tricky at first, but the accreditation manual is very clear, and after a few scoring sessions, organizations should be able to score themselves without any trouble. Here are examples of the categories:

Category A

This category is related to structural requirements, such as policies or plans. They either exist or they do not. This is a "yes" or "no" compliance question.

Example: IM.6.10, EP 1: Only authorized individuals make entries in the medical record.

Category B

This category may have structural or process requirements. There is also a qualitative component. The quality, adequacy, or comprehensiveness of your compliance must be self-evident. Follow good process design, which considers the following:

- The hospital's mission, values, and goals
- Patients' needs
- The use of currently accepted practices
- Current safety information and knowledge (e.g., sentinel event data, National Patient Safety Goals)
- Performance improvement results
- All components of the EP

Example: IM.6.10, EP 8: The hospital has a policy on the timely entry of information into the patient's medical record.

SCORING AND DECISION RULES

Category C

This category is based upon the number of times the hospital does not meet the EP. Measures of success (MOSs)—numerical or quantifiable measures related to an audit that determine whether an action was effective and sustained, or whether you are in compliance with the EP—are always required for Category C EPs. The (M) icon in the CAMH next to an EP indicates that an MOS is required along with a corrective action plan for any EP not in compliance.

Example: IM.6.30, EP 1 (M): The licensed independent practitioner (responsible for the patient) records the provisional diagnosis before the operation or other high-risk procedures.

Accreditation decisions

Accreditation decisions fall into six categories:

- Accredited
- Provisional accreditation
- Conditional accreditation
- Preliminary denial of accreditation
- Denial of accreditation
- Preliminary accreditation

See Figure 8.1 for a definition of each Joint Commission level of accreditation.

The accreditation decision becomes official once the organization submits the evidence of standards compliance (ESC) report after the on-site survey. This report details the actions the organization has taken to bring itself into compliance with standards or clarifies why it believes that it was already in compliance with the recommended findings. For any EP that requires a MOS, make sure to include the measure in your response.

CHAPTER EIGHT

Figure 8.1

The Joint Commission's levels of accreditation

Accredited
The Joint Commission awards this level to hospitals that demonstrate compliance with all standards during the on-site survey or those that address all requirements for improvement in an evidence of standards compliance submitted to The Joint Commission within 90 days of the survey. *(Note: Effective January 1, 2006, the time frame to submit evidence of standards compliance will be reduced to 45 days.)*

Provisional accreditation
The Joint Commission awards this designation to hospitals that show an acceptable level of overall standards compliance. However, the hospital hasn't successfully addressed all survey requirements for improvement (evidence of standards compliance) within specified time frames or hasn't achieved the appropriate level of sustained compliance based on a measure-of-success result.

Conditional accreditation
The Joint Commission awards this level of accreditation to hospitals that don't demonstrate substantial compliance with the standards (between two and three standard deviations from the mean number of requirements for improvement) or has met another decision rule for conditional accreditation. Organizations that receive this designation must undergo an on-site follow-up survey.

Preliminary denial of accreditation
The Joint Commission awards this level of accreditation to hospitals that have a high count of "not compliant" standards at the time of survey (more than three standard deviations above the mean number of requirements for improvement) or has met another decision rule for preliminary denial of accreditation. Hospitals can appeal the decision before The Joint Commission makes a formal determination to deny accreditation. It's worth appealing the decision, because The Joint Commission notes in its explanation of this accreditation level that the appeal process may also result in a decision other than denial of accreditation.

Denial of accreditation
The Joint Commission officially denies the hospital accreditation status. The hospital has no more opportunities to have its case reviewed or appealed.

Preliminary accreditation
The Joint Commission awards this level of accreditation to hospitals that demonstrate compliance with selected standards in the first of two surveys under Option 1 of the Early Survey Policy.

Source: The JCAHO Survey Coordinator's Handbook, Sixth Edition. *Copyright 2004, HCPro, Inc.*

At the end of the on-site survey

At the conclusion of the on-site survey, the facility will know exactly what the accreditation decision is and which standards (if any) require an ESC report. There are no longer any surprises: The ESC will be due 45 calendar days after the survey.

After the ESC is completed and any measures of success audited for four months, the process begins again—in fact, it should never stop. Remember that an aim of the new accreditation process is 100% compliance all the time and that processes and systems are continuously in place to provide quality patient care and safety.

CHAPTER 9

National Patient Safety Goals and other hot topics for ongoing records review

The National Patient Safety Goals (NPSGs) present special compliance and documentation opportunities (or challenges) for organizations. They are a major part of the on-site surveys, and The Joint Commission expects 100% compliance with them.

Because several of the goals require documentation in the medical record, they are important topics for ongoing records review. In addition, some of the tried and true "hot topics" for documentation, such as the preprocedure history and physical (H&P) and postoperative progress note, continue to be problems. This chapter will provide information related to both topics and give you ways to incorporate these important survey agenda items into your ongoing records review process.

NPSGs and other patient safety requirements

There are several NPSGs and other patient safety requirements that draw special attention to documentation in the medical record. Although for some of these goals surveyors will base judgments on observation and The Joint Commission does not necessarily require compliance with the goals to be entered in the record, a well-documented medical record can save headaches at survey time. In addition—and, perhaps, more important—communication among caregivers is essential to patient care and safety, and the medical record is the primary tool used for such communication.

That's why these patient safety goals fall into the category of improving communication. Several of these goals have become elements of performance (EPs) in the "Management of Information" (IM) chapter of the *Comprehensive Accreditation Manual for Hospitals* and are considered just as important as when they were listed specifically as NPSGs. They also are appearing on The Joint Commission's top list of noncompliant issues at the time of surveys.

Chapter Nine

Unapproved abbreviations

The Joint Commission is cracking down on unapproved use of abbreviations. IM.3.10, EP 2 requires organizations to standardize abbreviations, acronyms, and symbols throughout their facilities and to have a list of forbidden abbreviations, acronyms, and symbols. Concentrate on complying with the unapproved list, keep the list simple, and monitor it often. The unapproved abbreviations are ones that caregivers have used for a long time, and old habits are hard to break.

Standardized list

Because the EP refers to standardization, the organization should provide a reference list of acceptable abbreviations, acronyms, and symbols that hospital and medical staffs can access easily. Post the list on your organization's intranet, or use one of the reference books on the market that provide standardized abbreviations, acronyms, and symbols most often used in healthcare. Generally, the focus of your survey will be on the unapproved abbreviations, not the standardized ones, so spend your energy there.

Even though The Joint Commission's requirement for an unapproved list has been around for some time now, it is one of the highest noncompliant EPs. It has caused so much concern that The Joint Commission held a summit in 2004 to address the problem. After the summit, The Joint Commission clarified its compliance expectations for documentation of the organization's unapproved abbreviations. It made modifications to when it would require the unapproved list and how it would score findings. To outline the revisions to the requirements, the EP

- applies to all orders and all medication-related documentation (orders, transcription, medication administration records, progress reports, etc.).

- applies to preprinted forms that require 100% compliance and handwritten documentation that requires 90% compliance. Watch the latter, however, because the bar may soon be raised.

- does *not* apply to computer-generated forms or displays—at least for right now. It does apply to free text entries in the computer-generated forms.

NATIONAL PATIENT SAFETY GOALS AND OTHER HOT TOPICS FOR ONGOING RECORDS REVIEW

Steps to compliance

- Focus your efforts on the unapproved abbreviations, acronyms, and symbols; keep the list short and include The Joint Commission-required ones.

- Make it clear that everyone must comply, not just physicians.

- Conduct a review of all preprinted forms, and carefully monitor new ones before they are approved.

- Educate, educate, educate.

- Make review of records for unapproved abbreviations a standard part of your ongoing records review.

- Provide feedback (both good and bad) to hospital and medical staff departments.

- When reporting to the departments' leadership, be sure to provide reports by individuals making the unapproved abbreviation entries in the records. Generally, this is an individual issue that must be dealt with directly for improvement to occur.

- Require corrective action plans and target dates for resolutions.

- Get backing from senior management. The Joint Commission takes this seriously, so everyone in your organization must do so as well.

Best practice

The Joint Commission's Web site, *www.jointcommission.org*, provides examples of how organizations have tackled the unapproved abbreviations challenge. The following practices have also been very successful in organizations:

- One hospital held an abbreviations day (see Figure 9.1 for an example of a flier) to raise everyone's awareness of unapproved abbreviations. All departments that documented in the medical records were asked to review at least two records for unapproved abbreviations that day, and the information was trended and shared with the departments. It was also counted as an ongoing records review activity.

Chapter Nine

Figure 9.1

Unapproved abbreviations audit day flier

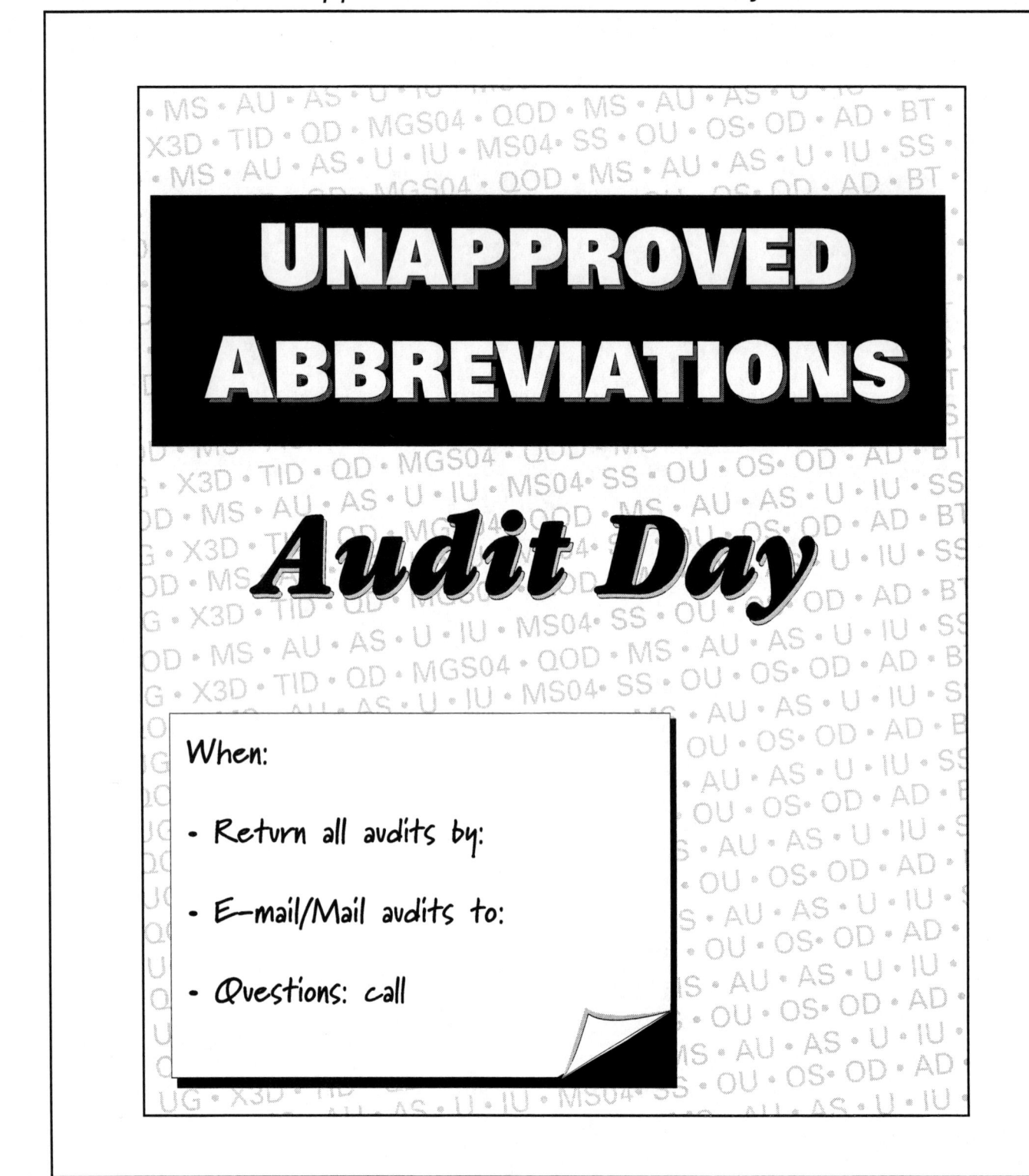

UNAPPROVED ABBREVIATIONS

Audit Day

When:

- Return all audits by:

- E-mail/Mail audits to:

- Questions: call

- Keep the list in front of everyone. Use the list as the image on mouse pads (a staff favorite), cups, pencils, or screen savers or attach it to hospital badges.

- Replace physicians' order tabs in open records on the units and outpatient areas with a red laminated tab that has the list on the back. When physicians write orders, they immediately see the list in front of them.

- Get the pharmacy involved. Take a hard line. Tell them not to fill orders containing unapproved abbreviations, acronyms, and symbols.

Figure 9.2

Patient safety goals/documentation audit tool

Goal/EP	Indictor	Indicator tool	Target	YTD	1st Q	2nd Q	3rd Q	4th Q
Improve accuracy of communication among caregivers	Unapproved abbreviations, acronyms, and symbols IM.3.10, EP 2	Chart audit	90% compliance/ paper records 100% compliance/ preprinted forms					
Improve accuracy of communication among caregivers	Verbal order "readback" IM.6.50, EP 4	Direct observation and chart audit	100% compliance					
Improve the accuracy of patient identification	Universal Protocol "time out" correct patient; correct site and side; correct procedure; correct patient position; correct x-rays displayed; verification of available implants, equipment, or special requirements	Direct observation and chart audit	100% compliance					
Timely reporting of critical test results and values	Reported to responsible provider within time frame set up by department	Department tracking log and chart audit	100% compliance					
Accurately and completely econcile medications across the continuum of care	2005: Develop process and documentation tools 2006: Medications reconciled at transfers and referrals	Chart audit	100% compliance					
Presurgical H&P, tests results, provisional diagnosis recorded before operation or procedure	H&P, tests results, provisional diagnosis on chart prior to operation or procedure IM.6.30, EP 1	Chart audit	100% compliance					
Operative reports dictated or written immediately after operation or procedure	Operative report dictated or written upon completion of the operation or procedure, before patient is transferred to the next level of care IM.6.30, EP 2	Operative/procedure report	100% compliance					
Postoperative progress note entered in medical record immediately after procedure	Postoperative progress note entered in record before patient is transferred to next level of care IM.6.30, EP 3	Chart audit	100% compliance					
Medication orders are written clearly and transcribed correctly	Orders for medications are legible and transcribed correctly MM.3.20	Medication orders received in the pharmacy	100% compliance					

Figure 9.3

Ongoing records review—open charts: Topic: Unapproved abbreviations

Information/indicator	Discharge date	MR#	MR#	MR#	MR#	MR#	MR#
1. U (for units)							
2. IU or iu							
3. QD or qd							
4. QOD or qod							
5. MS							
6. MSO4							
7. MgSO4							
8. AU							
9. AS							
10. AD							
11. OU							
12. OS							
13. OD							
14. BT							
15. HS or hs							
16. Ug							
17. SS or ss							
18. X3d							
19. Zero after decimal point							
20. No zero before decimal point							
21. No apothecary symbols							

Figure 9.4

Sample unapproved abbreviations ongoing review tool

REVIEWER			REVIEW DATE	
PATIENT NAME				
MR NUMBER			ACCT NUMBER	
ATTENDING PHYSICIAN			SURGEON	
OTHER PHYSICIANS				

DO NOT USE LIST	Intended Meaning	ABBREVIATION USED	LOCATION IN CHART	DATE AND TIME USED	PHYSICIAN OR STAFF MEMBER NAME	# OF TIMES USED	COMMENTS
MS	morphine sulfate						
MSO4	morphine sulfate						
MgSO4	magnesium sulfate						
OD or o.d. or od	once daily						
per os	orally						
Q.D. or q.d. or qd	once daily						
Q.O.D. or q.o.d. or qod	every other day						
qn	nightly or at bedtime						
qhs	nightly or at bedtime						
q6PM, etc.	every evening at 6:00 P.M.						
cc	cubic centimeters						
Trailing zero X.0 mg	X mg						
Lack of leading zero .X mg	0.X mg						
U	unit						
IU	international unit						

Source: Chester (SC) County Hospital. Reprinted in *Medical Records Briefing,* August 2004, with permission.

Chapter Nine

- Make findings from ongoing records review of unapproved abbreviations, acronyms, and symbols a part of the organization's quality report card. See Figure 9.2 for an example of a monitoring/reporting tool. You can include other troublesome documentation topics, as well.

Figures 9.3 and 9.4 provide review tools specifically used to monitor unapproved abbreviations, acronyms, and symbols. Your organization must determine what works. It may have to use several different approaches, but compliance must be the result of this ongoing records review activity.

Verbal/telephone order readback and verification

When verbal/telephone orders are not clearly understood and documented in the medical record or computer, mistakes can and do occur. For that reason, IM.6.50, EP 4 requires a process for taking verbal or telephone orders or for receiving critical test results that require a verification "readback" of the complete order or test result by the person receiving the order or test result. Although you can monitor this EP by observing the process, nothing works better than documenting it in the medical record. The hard part is making sure you are in compliance, which will require ongoing records review.

A clear understanding of this EP will go a long way toward compliance. The person taking the order (or receiving critical test results) must write it down and read it back to the person giving the order, and the person providing the information must verify that the order or test results are correct. The person receiving the information documents in the record that the information is verified and correct. To document, enter "RB/V"—for "read back/verified"—in the record beside the order or test results. Although documentation in the record is not required, it is best practice.

Steps to compliance

These steps are not much different from steps to compliance used for unapproved abbreviations:

- Provide a clear definition of the EP and place it and the process in an organizationwide policy.

- Continually educate, monitor, and trend both good and bad compliance.

- Provide feedback and expect correction where noncompliance exists.

- Take a no-tolerance stand on this NPSG. If the medical staff balk at verifying the order, refuse to take it.

National Patient Safety Goals and other hot topics for ongoing records review

- Stand behind your staff. And remember this applies to all caregivers receiving verbal/telephone orders and critical test values.

Best practice

If you do not already require documentation of the process, do so now. Audit both by observation and as part of ongoing records review.

Universal Protocol

Compliance with the "time out" continues to be a documentation challenge for organizations.

The Universal Protocol requires a preoperative verification process, surgical site- and side-marking process, and a "time out" or a pause immediately before the surgery/procedure begins so that the entire operating room (OR) team can agree to the following:

- Correct patient
- Correct site and side
- Correct procedure
- Correct patient position
- Correct x-rays displayed appropriately and verification of available implants, equipment, or special requirements

Best practice

Even if the site and side do not have to be marked, operations and procedures should include the "time out" process. The review for compliance with the Universal Protocol is a job for the OR staff that should be done at the time of the operation or procedure. Constant reminders of the process are a good idea, and Figure 9.5 provides a flier that you can post in all operative or procedure areas.

Critical test values

Although the laboratory has probably been performing this process for a long time, this 2005 NPSG requires expanding your list of critical test results and values to be monitored and assessed for timely reporting and receipt. When appropriate, the goal requires organizations to measure, assess, and take action regarding the timely reporting and receipt by the responsible licensed caregiver of critical tests

CHAPTER NINE

Figure 9.5

Universal Protocol for preventing wrong site, wrong procedure, wrong person surgery™

Applicable to invasive procedures in all settings

Wrong-site, wrong-procedure, wrong-person surgery can be prevented. The Universal Protocol is intended to achieve that goal. It is based on the consensus of experts from the relevant clinical specialties and professional disciplines and is endorsed by more than 40 professional medical associations and organizations.

1. PREOPERATIVE VERIFICATION PROCESS
   - ❐ Site/procedure verified with schedule, physician order, consent, and patient/patient representative

2. SURGICAL SITE MARKING
   - ❐ WHEN: Right/left, multiple structures or level

   - ❐ HOW: Physician initials site with approved skin marker, which must be visible after prep and drape

   - ❐ WHO: Surgeon/physician/radiologist with patient or patient representative

3. "TIME OUT" immediately BEFORE STARTING PROCEDURE
   - ❐ Involves entire team using active communication

   - ❐ Should indicate the following was validated:
     - Correct patient
     - Correct site and side
     - Correct procedure
     - Correct patient position
     - Correct x-rays displayed appropriately and verification of available implants, equipment, or special requirements

   - ❐ Fail-safe model: "NO GO" unless all agree

   - ❐ Verification and "time out" will be performed for all invasive procedures regardless of marking requirements, including those not involving a site mark—except in an emergency—if the risks outweigh the benefits

results and values. For example, radiology, cardiology, pulmonary, and obstetrics (fetal heart monitoring) should identify test results and values that fall into the critical category. It will be smart to keep the list as short as possible, but do not compromise patient care.

Best practice

The Massachusetts Coalition for the Prevention of Medical Errors (Massachusetts Coalition) has done some excellent work in this area. Its best practice guidelines[1] suggest that each organization should identify the following when tackling this topic:

- *Which* tests are critical to report
- The *time frames* for the process
- *To whom* the results should go
- *To whom* the results should go when the ordering provider is not available
- *How to* notify the responsible provider 100% of the time

Best practice indicates that you should develop a policy that identifies the above bullet points and put in place a process for monitoring timely outcomes. The departments and nursing are key players in the monitoring process, and the use of computer-generated reports will help make the process easier. The following list illustrates what should be included in a computer-generated report for radiology:

- MR#
- Exam code
- Check-in date/time
- Exam stop date/time
- Exam read date/time
- Exam typed date/time
- Release date
- Exam called date/time
- Recipient

Figure 9.6 provides an example of a radiology department policy. The laboratory's policy would be more specific because it has predefined high and low critical test values.

CHAPTER NINE

Figure 9.6

Policy and procedure

Policy #:	Originator (title):
Hospital:	Origination date:
Administrative approval:	Latest review/revision:
Administrative title:	Division/Imaging department:

Subject: Receiving and reporting critical test results

Purpose:
To ensure timely and reliable communication of critical test results.

Policy:
Critical test results are defined as any imaging procedure ordered as a "call report" by the ordering physician or any condition or finding determined by the interpreting radiologist as requiring immediate intervention for treatment.

Outpatient results will be called to the ordering physician's office. Inpatient results will be called to the patient's floor. ER discrepancies or findings deemed urgent by the interpreting radiologist will be called to the ER.

Procedure:

1. Critical test results will be communicated by imaging staff to a licensed clinician at the locations defined above.

2. Imaging staff will request read-back verification.

3. The licensed clinician receiving the results will read back the information and, whenever possible, will document the results in the appropriate patient record.

4. Imaging staff will document who communicated the results, the name of the licensed clinician who received the results, and the date and time of the communication in the radiology information system for the corresponding imaging study.

5. Reporting of the timeliness of the communication of critical test results will be accomplished via the radiology information system and results will be reported as a part of the imaging QPI indicators. The timeliness of reporting will be measured and assessed, and appropriate action will be taken as needed to make improvements.

Accurately and completely reconcile medications across the continuum of care

This is a tough but important NPSG, and The Joint Commission gave hospitals until 2006 to get in full compliance with it. It requires you to develop a process for obtaining and documenting, with the patient's help, a complete list of the patient's current medications upon admission (inpatient and outpatient) to the organization. The process also must include a comparison of the medications the organization provides to those on the list. And a complete list of the patient's medications must be communicated to the next provider of service for referrals and transfers to another setting, service, practitioner, or level of care within or outside of the organization.

Note that The Joint Commission expanded this goal for 2007: Hospitals must also provide to the patient the complete list of his or her medications on discharge from the facility.

Steps to compliance

This is a tall order, but one that was long in coming and completely in keeping with patient care and safety. The Massachusetts Coalition has also done work in this area, and you can access its Web site for more information (*www.macoalition.org*). Hospitals should begin to improve their processes for obtaining a current list of patient medications when patients arrive at the hospital and develop a process for communicating medication information to the next provider of care. Figure 9.7 provides samples of documentation tools to use for these purposes.

Best practice

Incorporate this process into your ongoing records review to ensure compliance. You can do so by developing a collaborative approach between nursing and pharmacy.

New goals added for 2007

Two new patient safety goals have been added for 2007. These include the following:

- Encourage patients' active involvement in their care as a patient safety strategy. Educate patients and families about methods available to report concerns related to care, treatment, and services, and encourage them to report concerns about safety.

- Identify safety risks inherent in the organization's patient population (i.e., patients at risk for suicide).

Best practice

Although there are no specific requirements for documentation in the medical records, make sure that these goals are reflected in assessments and reassessments within the medical record. It will be important to include them as part of ongoing record reviews in 2007 to validate compliance.

Figure 9.7

Medication reconciliation form

Patient name				Room number			
Medical record				Date of birth			
Allergies				Sex			
Account number							
Physician							
Active medications							
Continue	Discontinue	Change	Rx#	Description	Frequency	Start date	Stop date
Inactive medications							
Continue	Discontinue	Change	Rx#	Description	Frequency	Start date	Stop date

Physician signature/date:
Nurse signature/date:
Nurse signature/date:

Other hot topics

Other age-old topics continue to pop up on the lists of most frequently cited standards and EPs:

- H&Ps
- Operative and other high-risk procedure reports
- Postoperative progress notes
- Delinquent medical records
- Legibility

Delinquent medical records and legibility are still challenges for hospitals and top on the list for surveyors. All five topics should be standard items on your ongoing record review list. See Figure 9.2 for a tool to use in monitoring these high hitters.

H&P

IM.6.30, EP 9, requires that organizations record presurgical H&Ps before the operation or procedure.

Best practice

1. You will need a gatekeeper to ensure compliance. Do not allow the operation or procedure to proceed without the H&P and other information listed in the EP.

2. Use a short-form H&P for ambulatory cases. See Figure 9.8 for an example of an ambulatory H&P.

3. Have the medical staff define the minimum content, such as plan of care; past history as appropriate to the operation or procedure; and examination of heart, lungs, and mental status.

4. Make this topic part of your ongoing records review.

Operative and other high-risk procedure reports

IM.6.30, EP 2, calls for organizations to dictate or write operative and other high-risk procedure reports immediately after an operative or other high-risk procedure record.

Figure 9.8

Outpatient history and physical report

Hospital name (Patient label)

Outpatient history and physical report
Pertinent history (as appropriate to the patient's condition)

_____

_____

_____

Physical examination	Normal	Abnormal	If abnormal, explain below
1. Mental status			
2. Heart			
3. Chest/lungs			

	Normal	Abnormal	Deferred	If abnormal, explain below
4. Abdomen				
5. HEENT				
6. Neurological				
7. Lymph glands				
8. Neck				
9. Breasts				
10. Genitalia/vaginal				
11. Rectal				
12. Musculoskeletal				
13. Skin				
14. Other				

Anesthesia assessment and plan of care

Assessment	Plan of care
Previous problem(s) with sedation and/or anesthesia? No If yes, describe: _____	Local Moderate sedation Moderate sedation with local anesthesia If general, see anesthesia record

Medications: See physician orders   Yes   No

Principal/preoperative diagnosis:
_____
_____

Comorbid conditions:
_____
_____

Course of action planned: _____
_____

Physician signature: _____ **Date:** _____

Best practice

1. Have a clearly defined medical staff rule/regulation or policy related to this EP. The Joint Commission has defined "immediately" as "upon completion of the operation or procedure, before the patient is transferred to the next level of care."[2] Use this definition in your policy.

2. Keep close tabs on offenders. Report back to department chairs for corrective action.

Postoperative progress notes

IM.6.30, EP 3, requires organizations to enter the postoperative progress note into the medical record immediately after the procedure.

Best practice

1. Use a preprinted form (see Figure 9.9) or a stamp.

2. Identify where electronic output provides the postoperative progress note. For example, check your cardiac systems. If the information is electronically generated, you may not need the postoperative note.

3. Have the OR make these steps part of its ongoing records review.

Delinquent medical records

Chapter 5 provides information and best practices related to delinquent medical records. Here are a few more tips to help with this age-old problem:

- Regularly notify physicians of their incomplete and delinquent records
- Process discharged records in a timely manner
- Consistently apply the rule to all physicians
- Promote timely records completion as a quality of care and safety issue, not as a compliance issue
- Include timeliness as part of your ongoing records review

Chapter 11 provides a case study about one hospital's success with timely documentation.

Figure 9.9

Postoperative progress note

Hospital name: (Patient label)

Postoperative progress note (written immediately after surgery, before the patient goes to the next level of care)

Procedure(s) performed: _____

Name of primary surgeon: _____
Assistant(s): _____

Findings: _____

Technical procedures used: _____

Specimens removed: _____

Estimated blood loss: _____

Postoperative diagnosis: _____

Physician signature/date: _____

Legibility

This is a difficult area to tackle, but some hospitals have had success in improving legibility of their medical records. The following ideas represent best practice.

- Use preprinted orders for medications. Check boxes and fill-in orders for rates, doses, and routes can go a long way toward legible orders for medications. See Figure 9.10 for an example of a template.

- Consider promoting a state law that addresses legibility requirements for medical records. Two states, Florida and Washington, have this type of law.

- Develop a legibility policy to clarify expectations for legibility. See Figure 9.11 for a sample.

- Use a keyboard with computerized physician order entry, a stylus and personal data assistant (PDA) or a Palm Pilot device, or voice recognition software.

- Cut out bits of poor documentation, blow them up, and post them in the health information management (HIM) department. Have physicians and other hospital staff guess the authors.

- Involve the pharmacy in identifying legibility problems. Whenever the pharmacist has to have an order clarified because of illegible documentation, have the pharmacy staff send a copy of the order to the HIM director for tracking and trending. Report the data to the medical staff and nursing leadership.

- Use electronic signatures to sign off on reports.

- Conduct "legibility rounds," and rate documentation on a scale of 1–5, with 1 being illegible and 5 being very legible. Focus on the 1's first and then on the 2–4 group.

- Set up the electronic health record system.

CHAPTER NINE

Figure 9.10

Physician's preprinted orders

PHYSICIAN'S PREPRINTED ORDERS

(label)

(Physician name/group)

Date & time			
Diagnosis/procedure information	Procedure:	Condition stable fair serious critical	
Vital signs: ❏ unit routine ❏ hourly ❏ q 2 hrs. ❏ q 4 hrs. ❏ q 1 hr. for 4 hrs. then q 4 hrs. or unit routine ❏ Call physician for: ❏ P < 50 or > 110; ❏ BP > 10 mm Hg difference; ❏ decreased LOC; ❏ resp. distress			

Activity:

Diet:

Preop orders:

Nursing:

Labs:	❏ STAT	❏ in a.m.	❏ at ____:____
Diagnostics:	❏ STAT	❏ in a.m.	❏ at ____:____

Other:

IV:

Date & time	Drug (Generic name)	Dose concentration must be noted if dose is volume	Route	Frequency	Indications/special instructions
	Physician signature:				
	RN signature:				

Figure 9.11

Sample legibility policy

Purpose:
1. To define "illegible documentation" in a medical record.
2. To provide a framework for hospital and medical staff in determining legibility of all documentation in the medical record by all care providers.
3. To establish the mechanism for review of relevant information from the ongoing records review process and pharmacy interventions addressing illegible entries.

Applicability:
1. This policy is applicable to all healthcare documentation within the medical record, including nursing notes, progress notes, consultation records, physician orders, treatment records, etc.

Definitions:
1. Illegible—Very difficult or impossible to read by at least two professionals due to the entry being poorly written or printed.
2. Pharmacy intervention—Process by which a pharmacist or nurse initiates a phone call/contact with the prescribing practitioner to clarify a medication order.

Procedure:
1. Medical records review
   a. As per the medical record review policy, a 100% retrospective review of medical records will be performed by the medical record documentation review team, which consists of medical record coders assigned to review and code medical records for appropriate reimbursement.
   b. Legibility of medical record entries will be the key indicator during the medical record review.
   c. Any entry that cannot be read or interpreted during the review process is referred to the medical record committee for further evaluation. If the committee is unable to read or interpret the documentation, a letter from the committee is sent to the author in question, identifying the illegible entry. If after three consecutive monthly notifications the author does not improve, the issue is then referred to the respective department chair for further corrective action.
   d. Department chair, with the assistance of the director of health information management, will monitor the provider's progress over a 30-day period. If there is no significant improvement, the provider will be mandated to contract with a handwriting

CHAPTER NINE

Figure 9.11

Sample legibility policy

remediation consultant. If no further improvement has been made 30 days after working with the consultant, the provider will be directed to use available technologies offered by the hospital to document in the medical record.

2. Pharmacy interventions for clarification of illegible orders
   a. Pharmacy interventions will be recorded, aggregated, and analyzed, and appropriate action plans will be established by the director of health information management (medical records).
   b. Aggregated reports from pharmacy interventions will be reported monthly to the medical record committee.

3. Illegible medication and procedure orders
   a. Medication orders that are illegible, unclear, or incompletely written will not be carried out until clarified.
   b. The individual who wrote the original order will be contacted. If he or she is not available, then the covering practitioner will be contacted.
   c. Illegible orders that require an intervention will be entered into the MEDITECH Pharmacy Patient Intervention Module. A summary of the intervention will be generated in MEDITECH and reviewed by the medical record committee.

Aggregate data will be presented to the medical record committee, along with any appropriate action plans. This data will include legibility results.

The findings of the medical record committee are reported to the credentials committee and incorporated as part of the physician's credential file.

Process Cycle Information
Review Cycle Information
Reader Cycle Information

References:
Comprehensive Accreditation Manual for Hospitals; Institute for Safe Medication Practice (ISMP); Quarterly Action Agenda Institute for Safe Medication Practice; Whitepaper on Electronic Prescribing; 2000 American Society of Health-System Pharmacists (ASHP).

Source: South Shore Hospital. Reprinted with permission.

Best practice

A relatively new concept says that time pressure, not bad handwriting, leads to illegibility.

Therefore, to combat illegible orders, Robert Marder, MD, practice director of quality and patient safety for The Greeley Company, a division of HCPro, advocates STAR, a technique he adapted with Performance Improvement International (PII) to help combat errors in healthcare (see the related case study in Chapter 11).

PII has identified time pressure as one of the major sources of human error in multiple industries. That is, when people are under pressure, they make mistakes or do not carry out tasks as well as they ordinarily would. Marder thought about this concept as he worked on error reduction with medical staffs in hospitals. He thought that by addressing the root cause of time pressure (the fundamental cause of error), there would be a greater chance of improving legibility instead of trying to improve penmanship, which would decline under time pressure.

Marder himself is a perfect example—he admits to having terrible handwriting. But when his 10-year-old-daughter asked him whether he could ever write legibly, he showed her that he could. He simply slowed down and was patient, and he wrote a sentence that anyone can read. "It's not beautiful," he admits, "but it's legible."

The STAR technique—which stands for Stop, Act, Think, Review—encourages physicians to slow down at crucial times. The concept was originally developed to help seventh grade students with math tests, based on the fact that even though the students might know the right answer, they might write the wrong answer because they are in a hurry. The students didn't like the approach, but the nuclear power industry successfully adopted it to help reduce operator errors.

The fundamental approach to STAR calls for a physician to do the following:

Stop or slow down for a second before doing a critical task (e.g., write an order or a note)
Think about the desired outcome (e.g., I want to write slowly to get a legible order)
Act to perform the task in a way that will achieve the outcome (e.g., write more slowly to make sure the order can be read)
Review to make sure the desired outcome was achieved (e.g., look over the order to make sure I can read it)

Chapter Nine

"People who have the problem with legibility usually realize it. In fact, most illegible orders are not legible to physicians who wrote them. So the review process is basically the self-checking. If the order is legible, they are done. If it's not legible to them, they go back and fix it right there and then. It saves them time because they don't get a call from someone later about it because someone couldn't read it. And it improves patient safety," Marder explains.

To successfully implement the STAR technique at your organization, Marder says that you'll need the support of medical staff leaders who are committed to sitting down with physicians and going through STAR training. Although training physicians in groups will work, Marder says it's best to have one-on-one training sessions with problematic physicians.

"This technique is best for the medical staff that wants to deal with legibility but doesn't think that strategies to improve penmanship are successful," Marder says. "If your medical staff is not engaged in solving the problem, then it won't be successful."

Chapter 11 and the CD-ROM include case studies related to legibility: The CD-ROM features one from a previous edition of this book and Chapter 11 has a new success story related to the STAR technique. Both refute the saying that "you can't teach an old dog new tricks." Whatever technique you use, remember that legibility is the responsibility of anyone making entries in the medical record, and monitoring should be part of your ongoing records review process.

Other documentation challenges

EPs, such as PC.13.120, EP 2 (H&P entered in record within 24 hours of admission), and PC.8.10, EP 1 (pain assessment), continue to be documentation challenges. Including these topics as part of your ongoing records review will be an important step toward ensuring compliance.

This book has offered several examples of review tools for H&P compliance. Best practice indicates that those organizations that review for H&Ps at the point of care and expect 100% compliance achieve the best results. Figure 3.1 provides an example of a tool to use for review of the timeliness and quality of H&Ps. See Figure 9.12 for a tool to use when reviewing documentation for pain.

Figure 9.12

Medical record review tool for pain management

UNIT _____ DATE _____

STANDARD	P = PRESENT A = ABSENT N/A = NOT APPLICABLE	1 P / A / N/A MR#	2 P / A / N/A MR#	3 P / A / N/A MR#	4 P / A / N/A MR#	5 P / A / N/A MR#	6 P / A / N/A MR#	7 P / A / N/A MR#
	Pain management							
	1. Admission assessment							
	Use of pain scale on initial assessment							
	a. Documented intensity of pain using 1–10 pain scale							
	b. Documented location of pain							
	c. Documented duration of pain							
	d. Documented pain relieved by:							
	e. Documented type of pain							
	If score greater than 4, was treatment initiated?							
	a. Pharmacologic?							
	b. Nonpharmocologic?							
	c. Pain reevaluated after 1 hour?							
	2. Daily Reassessment							
	Reassessment includes a patient's response to care							
	a. Pain reassessed daily							
	b. Documented using 1–10 scale							
	c. Interventions noted							
	d. Response to interventions noted							
	3. Pain assessment completed on:							
	a. PCA flow sheet							
	b. Narcotic flow sheet							
	c. Postprocedure record							
	4. Care of patients							
	a. Care planning considers patient specific pain management needs, age-specific needs, severity level of condition, and impairment							
	b. Clinical observations, including the results of therapy							
	c. Monitoring of a medication's effect on the patient includes assessment based on collective observations, including the patient's own perception of its effect on pain							
	5. Education of patients							
	a. The patient is educated about pain and effective pain management, as needed							
	6. Discharge planning							
	a. Discharge instructions in regard to pain management							
	7. Postoperative monitoring of pain							
	a. Pain intensity and quality is documented							

Chapter Nine

Whether the issues are specific to your organization or are on The Joint Commission's Top 10 list, include the critical topics at the top of your list of ongoing record review indicators. And expect compliance. Consistent monitoring, assessing, and reporting will yield good results in the end.

A look ahead to 2008

In December 2007 The Joint Commission released for review a list of goals and requirements that will be considered for potential inclusion in the 2008 NPSGs. Should these be accepted, the new goals would require hospitals to

- improve recognition and response to changes in a patient's condition
- reduce the risk of postoperative complications for patients with obstructive sleep apnea
- prevent patient harm associated with healthcare worker fatigue
- prevent catheter misconnections

Other potential requirements include requiring organizations to investigate and initiate planning for the use of technology to assist with patient identification and to reduce the likelihood of patient harm associated with the use of anticoagulation therapy.

The use of technology to assist with patient identification has some possible ramifications for HIM departments, if this NPSG is accepted.

Joint Commission NPSG requirement 1A, which requires the use of two patient identifiers when treating patients, has a potential new implementation expectation requiring hospitals to investigate and plan to implement new technology, such as barcoding or a radio-frequency identification system. When investigating a system, the organization should determine

- what kind of system to use
- a timeline for evaluating and implementing the new technology
- the scope of the implementation
- what resources would be needed to implement the system
- an assessment of risk stemming from a new system

This is a new version of a previous proposed goal, which required that hospitals establish a barcoding system for patient identification. That goal received a lot of attention in years past, especially because it included firm dates for establishing and using the system. The proposed 2008 goal offers no timeline, but it does require hospitals to develop their own schedule to implement this change.

Note that these goals are still up for public comment and are not final for 2008.

Endnotes

1. *www.macoalition.org/initiatives.shtml*
2. Joint Commission on Accreditation of Healthcare Organizations, 2007 *Comprehensive Accreditation Manual for Hospitals*, Oakbrook Terrace, IL: The Joint Commission.

CHAPTER 10

One hospital system's experience with two unannounced Joint Commission surveys

The author's hospital system experienced two unannounced Joint Commission on-site surveys in 2006. Therefore, it seemed appropriate to include in the fifth edition of *Ongoing Records Review* an overview of these experiences. You can find a summary of the survey at the end of the chapter.

In addition, this chapter provides tips, tools, and strategies to assist organizations with their own unannounced surveys.

The Joint Commission facilitator's role

The system's two hospitals were due to be surveyed in 2006. Unfortunately, the surveys did not occur at the same time, nor were they conducted with the same surveyors as in the past.

Preparing for and maintaining momentum for multiple hospitals in a system can be a challenge. This is even more true if one or several hospitals are surveyed early in the year and other hospitals have to wait until later.

The best method of recognizing these challenges and meeting them is through a Joint Commission coordinator. His or her role should include overseeing, delegating, and assisting in the following activities:

- Regular performance of tracers
- Review of medical records for compliance with standards
- Keeping documents up-to-date
- Orienting new employees to The Joint Commission survey process
- Motivating other employees

Chapter Ten

The longer staff have to wait for a survey to occur, the harder it is to keep momentum going. Therefore, The Joint Commission facilitator must be both the cheerleader and the educator until all surveys are completed within the organization—and continually thereafter.

Preparing for the survey

Even though organizations should ideally be prepared at all times, there are many specific things a hospital can do in the year of an unannounced survey. As stated in previous sections of this book, education, mock surveys, and patient tracers with a focus on the National Patient Safety Goals (NPSG) are a given. It is vital to make sure that staff who are directly responsible for patient care are comfortable with the survey process, because they will be the ones with whom the surveyors will talk.

Of course, complete, accurate, and timely medical records will make all the difference in a successful survey. The organization's periodic performance review is an excellent tool to identify opportunities for improvement.

Most important, you have to start preparing *now*. Keep the tracers going all the time, and maintain a calendar and a process for performing them. Good data from tracers is important because it allows you to keep your managers accountable for making corrections.

10 tips to help prepare for an unannounced Joint Commission survey

Here are some proven tips to help you prepare for an unannounced Joint Commission survey:

1. **Establish a Joint Commission oversight team (or activate an existing one).** This group will be responsible for making sure all the steps for preparation described above are completed and reported. This team should also ensure that any noncompliant issues are resolved.

2. **Assign a representative to check the organization's secured Web site (The Joint Commission Connect™ link at *www.jointcommission.org*) on a regular basis.** It is critical that this person check the Web site sharply at 7 a.m. Monday through Friday, because on the morning of survey, a notice will appear, along with surveyor identification information, that the unannounced survey will occur that day. Surveyors come knocking on your door around 7:45 a.m., so it's smart to be prepared and give yourself as much advance notice as possible.

3. **Identify staff who will greet the surveyors.** These might be volunteers or security guards who will require some education on proper surveyor-greeting protocol. For example, whoever will greet the surveyors will need to know that he or she must request identification, know whom to call, and know where to take the surveyors upon arrival.

4. **Establish a call tree, publish it, and make it available to your entire staff.** Your organization must have a well-placed plan to ensure that everyone is notified on the morning of an unannounced survey. A backup list is also important, because chances are someone will not be there on the days of the survey. (Figure 10.1 provides an example of an instruction sheet and call tree.)

5. **Assign someone to accompany the surveyors on their rounds.** Generally a two-person team is best. Most surveyors will request that the hospital not send along a large entourage when they conduct tracers. It's a good idea to match up a clinical and a nonclinical guide. It is also important that this two-person team

    - know their way around the organization
    - know managers of each department for introduction purposes
    - split their duties accordingly: One person should act as the guide, and the other should act as a scribe to take notes, retrieve requested information, etc.

6. **Establish a location for the "command center" and designate staff to man the phones.** It is a good idea to give surveyors one telephone number to call if they need information such as policies, etc.

7. **Provide a workroom for the surveyors.** Include lunch for the surveyors each day. Surveyors will need a space to review documents, plan their agendas, and determine final survey results.

8. **Identify the person who will coordinate receipt of the documents requested for the documents review.** Generally, this is The Joint Commission facilitator. He or she will make sure all documents are in place, identified, and kept updated. See Figure 10.2 for an example of a cover sheet that can be used for each document notebook.

Chapter Ten

Figure 10.1

The Joint Commission unannounced survey instruction sheet

Hospital name

7:00 a.m.—Monday–Friday
Identify the person who checks the The Joint Commission Connect™ Web site Monday–Friday.
1. Person calls administrator and the nursing supervisor on duty.
2. Person who checks Web site e-mails "all users" that the surveyors are scheduled to arrive.
3. Nursing supervisor calls the information desks, the security guard, and the switchboard.
4. The switchboard announces (via overhead page) that "The hospital welcomes The Joint Commission surveyors who are at the hospital this morning."
5. The switchboard calls in order of priority*:

Primary call list	Secondary call list
Hospital to determine	Hospital to determine

8:45 a.m.—Information desks/security guards/administrative supervisor
Include information about where you expect the surveyors to arrive.

Information desk/security guards
There will be three or four surveyors, depending on whether the engineer comes on the first day. When the surveyors present, ask for their identification. They are accustomed to this question and will be expecting it. Direct the surveyors to have a seat and explain that you are calling the nursing supervisor to come escort them to the administrator's office.

Nursing supervisor
The nursing supervisor goes to the location of the surveyors and escorts them to the administrator's office.

* Primary and secondary call lists: Come to the hospital as soon as possible. Go to your office and someone will call you as you are needed. Names in **BOLD** go directly to administrator's office.

Figure 10.2

Sample cover sheet for requested Joint Commission documents

Title of document notebook/folder

Hospital: _____

Documents: _____

Data source: _____

Frequency of updates: _____

Person responsible for information: _____

Telephone number: _____

Backup person responsible for information: _____

Telephone number: _____

Format for the information: _____

_____ Electronic   _____ Printout

9. **Keep your documents well organized and up-to-date on the first morning of the survey.**
   Well-organized documents will result in fewer requests later. See Figure 10.3 for a list of required documents.

10. **Identify who will participate in the interviews, and practice with mock interviews.**
    The organization should be prepared for the following interview sessions, depending on the length of the survey:

    - Opening conference and orientation to the organization
    - Competence assessment process
    - Medical staff credentialing and privileging
    - Environment of care
    - *Life Safety Code®* building assessment
    - Leadership session
    - Medication management
    - Infection control
    - Data flow
    - Exit conference

It goes without saying that identification and publication of the locations for the sessions are also important.

An excellent resource for survey preparation is The Joint Commission's *Survey Activity Guides*, provided on the secured portion of The Joint Commission Web site (The Joint Commission Connect™). It has everything you need to know to be prepared for your unannounced survey. If you follow this guide, you can sit back and relax on the days of the survey.

Figure 10.4 provides a checklist tool to help you prepare for your unannounced survey.

The role of HIM in preparation

You may have noticed that there is no mention of closed record reviews and the role of the HIM director and staff. As noted in previous chapters, the HIM professionals and staff will continue to play a vital role in regard to ongoing record reviews and identification of opportunities for improvement in documentation. They can also serve as great Joint Commission facilitators, guides, and "command center" personnel.

Figure 10.3

Documents required for unannounced surveys

- 12 months of performance improvement data

- 12 months of infection control surveillance data

- Environment of care data, including statement of conditions and plans for improvement, management plans and annual evaluations, and 12 months of environment of care team meeting minutes

- Organizational chart

- Map of the organization

- List of departments, units, and services

- Census, clinic visits, and operating room schedules on days of survey to identify tracer patients

- Name of key contact person

- Priority focus process data: Provide performance improvement data, failure modes and effects analysis, and other data that addresses organization-specific priority focus areas

- Measures of success from periodic performance review action plan

- ORYX data

- Organ donation and procurement conversion rates (hospital only)

- Medical record delinquency data (hospital only)

- List of home visits for duration of survey (home health only)

* Reference: The Joint Commission Survey Activity Guide.

CHAPTER TEN

Figure 10.4

Joint Commission check-off preparedness list

Action item	Comments	Date complete
Identify oversight team and set meeting agenda		
Identify individual and backup to check Web site Monday–Friday, 7:00 a.m. EST		
Identify surveyor greeters for first morning and educate		
Call tree compiled and published		
Guides for surveyors identified and educated		
Command center location identified		
Command center staff identified and educated		
Identify workroom for surveyors		
Arrange for refreshments/lunches		
Identify documents coordinator		
Documents complete and updated		
Identify interview session attendees; provide guide to interviews; practice;		
Establish agenda for mock surveys and tracers; conduct mock surveys and tracers		
Establish education schedule*		

*Use formal education sessions, department meetings, intranet Web site.

Final words on preparation

Be ready all the time, but give special emphasis to preparation the year of your unannounced survey. A knowledgeable and passionate staff, focused on the quality of care they provide, coupled with physicians who take an active role in the care of their patients and the operations of the organization, will come across loud and clear to the surveyors. These, along with an accurate, timely, and legible medical record, will go a long way toward success.

At the conclusion of the survey

Everyone breathes a sigh of relief, and then the work begins again. If there are requirements for improvement, you must submit a response to the Jayco Web site within 45 days of notice of the final report. If measures of success (MOS) are required, an action plan and audit schedule must be approved by The Joint Commission. Your hospital then monitors for four months and submits its achieved goal to the Joint Commission. These are important action steps, and you should comply with them exactly as they are outlined. Full compliance with MOS must be accomplished within the four-month audit period.

Survey experience

Since the author's hospital system had been last surveyed in 2003, it was pretty certain that 2006 would bring an unannounced survey to its doors and that the two hospitals would be surveyed at different times during the year—which is exactly what happened.

Each day, the author monitored the secured portion of The Joint Commission Web site to see whether the survey was to occur. You only know the morning of the survey that surveyors are coming; this is why you have to check the Web site regularly. Usually the Web site says "no information available"; however, on this particular morning, we were alerted with the surveyors' names and pictures. You immediately know when today is the day.

The author was the first point of contact, and after seeing the prompt on the Web site, she contacted the administrator, the president of the system, the chief nurse executive, and the hospital switchboard. The call tree filtered down from there—the switchboard called people, the chief nursing executive's assistant called nurse managers, and staff made an overhead announcement: "We welcome the Joint Commission surveyors to our campus this week." The author also sent out an "all-users e-mail" to alert staff that the surveyors had arrived.

Chapter Ten

The survey team included an administrator, a nurse, a physician, and an engineer. The second facility was surveyed later in the year, and that survey team included a physician and a nurse. Despite the differences in hospital sizes, both surveys were similar in nature and followed the same agenda with a focus on patient tracers throughout the duration of the surveys. The first survey lasted four days, and the second survey was three days.

The engineer stayed for only one day to survey the environment of care and statement of conditions. The nurse, physician, and administrator stayed for the full four days. The surveyors are early risers and stayed every day from 8 a.m. to 5 p.m.

Preidentified staff greeted the surveyors at the door and helped get them settled in the appropriate conference room at the hospital. After the initial "meeting and greeting," the surveyors want to look at the organization's documents. It's important to have your documents in good order. Generally, this will reduce the number of documents requested later in the survey. After the surveyors review your documents, they begin the patient tracers, which consume the lion's share of the survey agenda.

The threads of the survey focused on the NPSGs, the organization's priority focus areas, and clinical service groups. The surveyors also conduct interviews throughout the agenda and validate or clarify what they observe during patient and system tracers.

Each morning, the surveyors required an inpatient census and operating room schedule. Patient tracers are identified, and then the surveyors and their guides talk with staff and patients. Generally, the first stops are at the inpatient units and the ancillary departments where the patient has been treated. The use of the medical record, whether paper, electronic, or a combination of both, is the tool used by all surveyors to identify the patient's path and identify which caregivers will be interviewed.

Areas of focus in the survey included the following:

- Assessments, to include the history and physical (and its update, if done prior to admission or outpatient surgery)

- Reassessments

- Pain management

- Operative reports and postoperative notes

- Legibility

- Management of medications, with an emphasis on review by the pharmacist or physician, storage (security), and orders that include indication for the medication prescribed

- NPSGs—see Chapter 9 for tips on compliance

- Disaster credentialing for those coming into the organization who are not on staff (with the revisions in 2007 to the "Medical Staff" chapter, be prepared for a heavy focus on this area)

A conference room that included tables, chairs, phones, computer hook-ups, and adequate working space was provided for the surveyors to work from each day. Here, they could come and go, confer with each other, and compare notes in complete privacy. Refreshments and lunch were provided each day.

A very special "plus" to the new survey process is the consultative approach the surveyors take in providing immediate feedback during the survey. Staff and leaders know every day any issues that have been identified during the tracers. Adequate opportunities exist to discuss with and ask questions of the surveyors. They are open about what they see, and they give you good feedback. Never be afraid to ask questions or challenge issues if you feel surveyors are on the wrong track. Developing a good rapport with the surveyors is a plus. A debriefing at the end of the day helps to keep the survey in perspective and gets the issues out on the table.

Of course you won't know until the last day exactly what the outcome will be. The surveyors put all their data into the computer, and that provides the final results.

Summary of the experience

The survey was not an added burden, although stress was a bit high throughout the system until the day finally arrived. The staff felt comfortable talking about their patients, and the surveyors recognized their enthusiasm for what they do best—take care of patients.

Chapter Ten

The surveyors were helpful. They provided helpful and constructive feedback and were willing to share good examples of forms and policies that they have collected during other surveys and that they consider best practice. Don't be afraid to ask for copies of these forms and policies, as the author found the surveyors willing to share. And don't be afraid to ask for advice on better ways to improve your processes. Surveyors have seen many organizations and have a good feel for what works best.

Overall, The Joint Commission unannounced survey is an excellent process—much better than the old methodology. The tracer methodology provides the "real picture" of what happens within the organization and whether processes are working well to provide quality and safe patient care.

More helpful tools

Some additional forms are included at the end of this chapter to help you prepare for Joint Commission unannounced surveys. They are as follows:

- Figure 10.5 provides some Joint Commission sample survey questions to help get your staff in the right frame of mind for what the surveyors may ask. It is not an all-inclusive list.
- Figure 10.6 provides a list of preparedness tips to distribute to your various departments.
- Figure 10.7 provides a leadership interview reference sheet. Distribute this to physicians, chief executive officers, and upper-level management to help them understand the surveyors' areas of focus.

Figure 10.5

The Joint Commission sample survey questions

Opening conference and orientation
1. What have you done on the conversion rate of organ donors?
2. Do you have any employed physicians?
3. How many physicians are on staff? How many are on the board? Does the chief of staff sit as an ex-officio member of the board?
4. Are medical records completely electronic?
5. Is there currently any new construction or remodeling going on within the hospital?
6. Where are you at with medication reconciliation?
7. Are all licensed independent practitioners credentialed the same as physicians or employees are?
8. What have you done to educate the staff on Accreditation Participation Requirement 17?
9. What are you doing to recruit nurses?
10. How are you working with schools/colleges to promote healthcare worker careers?
11. What are you doing within the state to address healthcare worker recruitment?
12. How do you ensure that staff are educated about patient safety goals?

Information requested for document review
- Contracts for dialysis and outside lab services, to ensure that the contracts addressed the need for them to meet The Joint Commission requirements
- Policy for credentialing emergency volunteer physicians in the case of a disaster
- Policy that outlines the process for requesting an outside focused peer review

Patient tracers

Blood bank
1. How do nurses get critical lab value information from the lab to the physician?

Dialysis
1. What types of patients do you care for here? What is your patient population? What health problems do you recognize within this population?
2. How does the doctor work here? Does he or she care for all the patients?
3. How often is tubing changed? How is equipment cleaned? How often are biohazard bags taken care of?
4. What brought this patient to dialysis? Why is he or she receiving dialysis?

Figure 10.5 (cont.)

The Joint Commission sample survey questions

5. How does the charge nurse in dialysis get the information about the patient for whom he or she is caring?
6. What do you think medication reconciliation means?
7. How long do the doctors have to sign verbal orders? Do doctors have to date and sign orders?
8. What is your process of patient education? Where is it documented that the patient or family verbalized or understood this process?

Respiratory therapy
1. How do you accomplish staff education?

PCA
1. Where is the patient education that you provide for patient care assistants (PCAs)?
2. Do staff know that they can contact The Joint Commission anytime with a complaint/concern and that there will be no retaliation from hospital management?
3. What have you done to increase safety in your department?
4. How are you competent to do this job? What classes or courses have you attended in the past year? Have you gone to any training outside the hospital?
5. What would you do if there was a fire in this room right now?

OR
1. Where are the exits in the operating room (OR)?
2. How do you prevent surgical fires?

Crash carts
1. What is the procedure to change out drawers? What are the meanings of the different colored locks?
2. How do you handle discrepancies from your medication dispensing system?

Pharmacy
1. How do you obtain and stock meds in the hospital?
2. How quickly are access codes eliminated?
3. Are any ad-mixed medications mixed outside the pharmacy? What is the process to ensure competency for nurses?

Figure 10.5 (cont.)

The Joint Commission sample survey questions

SDSU
1. What are the staffing ratios for your same day surgical unit (SDSU)?

Responding to a code
1. Who is involved in a code?
2. Who critiques the code?
3. Do you inform other units about the performance of the code?

Cath lab
1. Are you doing an airway assessment on each patient prior to the procedure?

Radiology
1. How is this area cleaned?
2. What is the process for bringing biopsies to the lab, and how are they logged?
3. How are peds patients managed in this area?

Physical therapy
1. Why is this patient here?
2. What is the patient's medical background?
3. Does this patient have advance directives?
4. Is patients' pain control noted as they're coming and going?
5. Where do you find patient identifiers?
6. What is included in morning report? Where do you give morning report?
7. What do you do if you can't read a signature?

Endoscopy
1. How are emergency meds handled?

Pediatrics
1. How does case management get involved over the weekend?

Data review
1. What things are you doing to improve pain management?
2. Do you have data showing improvement?

Figure 10.5 (cont.)

The Joint Commission sample survey questions

3. What have you done regarding a Failure Mode effects analysis?
4. What have you done regarding your Measures of Success?

Leadership survey
1. How do the board and medical staff participate in development of the system's strategic and management plans? What quality initiatives have you undertaken during the past year?
2. How do the leaders set priorities for the organization?
3. How do you use data to make improvements?
4. How are you involved in emergency planning?
5. How do you collect data and bring about consequences? How do you know you are achieving your objectives?
6. What do you do about outliers, and who brings those forward?
7. May we see your policy that outlines the process to obtain an outside focused review of a physician's chart, if needed?
8. How do you manage what is going on at your ambulatory sites (far away)? How is the management contract overseen?
9. Describe three or four concerns for both the nursing staff and medical staff.

Credentialing survey
1. When you hire a new person, what are the beginning credentialing steps?
2. What other competencies are done?
3. What do you do with an employee with a substance abuse problem?
4. How do you maintain licensure verification?

Infection control
1. Who is on your infection control (IC) committee?
2. What type of IC data do you look at?
3. What is the average length of time a Foley catheter is in?
4. Who helps you monitor hand hygiene?
5. Who is your committee chair? What is his or her specialty? How often does the committee meet?
6. Do you have good participation at your committee meetings?
7. Tell me about your PPD (TB skin test) program. How is the medical staff immunized?

Figure 10.6

Departmental preparedness tips

Assessments/reassessments
Every patient must be assessed for allergies, advance directive, pain, social and religious needs, discharge planning, falls, rehabilitation services, nutrition, and education regarding care and treatment. Documentation should be found in the medical record. Reassessments should occur at the change of shift.

History and physical reports
History and physical (H&P) must be in the medical record within 24 hours of admission or prior to any surgery. If the H&P was performed before admission or the day before outpatient surgery, you must write an update in the medical record, or document "no changes" on the H&P or progress note.

Postoperative progress note
Physicians must always document a postoperative progress note and dictate a full operative report **immediately** after the procedure/surgery.

Verbal and telephone orders
Verbal and telephone orders must be signed within 48 hours of when the order is given. Put a "sign here" tag on orders when you document them in the medical record.

Plan of care
The plan of care must be interdisciplinary and address the patient's needs as they are identified or occur.

Physician privileges
Enter your hospital-specific instructions on how to locate physicians' privileges to practice and perform surgery.

Audibility of alarms
Identify department that performs alarm tests when equipment is either repaired or has a Preventative Maintenance performed. Managers should have a routine process for checking the audibility of alarms such as call bells, bathroom bells, and bed alarms.

Figure 10.6 (cont.)

Departmental preparedness tips

Hand washing
Hands should be washed before and after entering a patient room, passing medication, and providing care and treatment.

Refrigerator
All refrigerators must be checked for proper temperature every day and logged on the temperature log. The log should be in view on the refrigerator door.

Nourishments
Patient nourishments should be kept separate from staff nourishments. Refrigerators should designate patient nourishments. Outdated food items should be discarded.

Shutting off the oxygen (O2) in the event of an emergency
Provide instruction on how this occurs, and a reference policy.

Environment
Patient care storage rooms, clean and dirty linen rooms, storage rooms, break rooms, etc. should all be neat and clean. Door should be closed at all times. All storage items should be 18 inches from the ceiling.

Medications
- Medications, crash carts, and medication carts must be secured at all times.
- Syringes and needles should never be left on tops of carts or in unsecured areas.
- Medications must NOT be expired.
- You should have a list of "look-alike" and "sound-alike" medications on your Pyxis machines and in other appropriate areas.

FMEA
Failure modes and effects analysis (FMEA) is an approach to identifying potential risk areas before they happen. *Provide an example of an FMEA here.*

Staffing effectiveness
- Staffing effectiveness data can identify issues that can occur when there is not enough staff; for example, weekend might identify an increase in falls.
- Managers should know their staffing effectiveness data and share with staff.

Figure 10.6 (cont.)

Departmental preparedness tips

Data

The use of data to improve patient care quality and safety is important. You should know how to use data to improve patient care quality and safety on your unit/department. **Examples** could be the use of patient and employee satisfaction data, performance improvement data, chart audits, measuring your timely reporting of critical tests values/results, etc.

Know the National Patient Safety Goals and practice them 100% of the time:

1. **Two identifiers**—name and date of birth; if DOB is not available, use medical record number. You must always check the name and DOB (or MR#) against a source.
2. **Reporting critical tests results/values** to the appropriate caregiver within two hours of receiving the information. You must have data to support compliance with the time frames for reporting to the caregiver.
3. **Read back and verify verbal and telephone orders and critical test results and values:** a) Document the order/results in the record; b) read back to the caregiver; c) caregiver verifies; d) document RB/V after order/critical test results/value.
4. **Universal Protocol includes the following:**
    - Preoperative checklist
    - Marking the site, if appropriate
    - Time out
5. **Hand washing:** Follow CDC guidelines.
6. **Audible alarms:** May sure alarms can always be heard and are tested regularly.
7. **Reconciling medications process includes**
    - a list of home medications
    - comparing list of home meds to current meds when patient changes level of care, when transferred, and at discharge
    - list of meds given to patient at discharge
8. **PROHIBITED abbreviations: DO NOT USE!**
9. **Look-alike/sound-alike medications:** Should be posted on Pyxis and other appropriate medication locations.
10. **Hand off:** Communication between caregivers when patients change levels of care, are transferred and discharged—there must be an opportunity to ask questions and receive clarification from one caregiver to the other.
11. **Standardized drug concentration:** Pharmacy and therapeutics committee reviews the hospital medication formulary to ensure standardization.
12. **IV pumps:** IV pumps assist with calculations and limit errors.

Chapter Ten

Figure 10.6 (cont.)

Departmental preparedness tips

13. **Labeling meds and medication containers:** Perioperative and procedural areas only.
14. **Reduce the risk of healthcare-associated infections:** Manage as sentinel events all identified causes of unanticipated deaths or major permanent loss of function associated with healthcare-associated infection.
15. **Reduce risk of harm from falls:** Assess, reassess, and take action.

Patient tracer

"Patient tracer" is the method the surveyors will used to conduct surveys. They will identify a patient's medical records and follow the patient's path through a hospitalization. This will include any outpatient areas where the patient entered or was treated. The surveyors will talk to the caregivers taking care of the patient.

Remember, in case of a fire:

R	Rescue	**P**	Pull
A	Alarm	**A**	Aim
C	Contain	**S**	Squeeze
E	Extinguish	**S**	Sweep

Figure 10.7

Joint Commission leadership interview reference sheet

Priority focus areas

Note: Each subsection below contains examples. Each hospital should develop its own.

Definition of priority focus areas (PFAs)
Processes, systems, or structures in a healthcare organization that significantly impact quality and safety of care. PFAs guide the assessment of standards components in relation to the patient tracer activities.

1. **Quality improvement expertise and activities:** Identifying issues and establishing priorities; developing measures; collecting data to evaluate status on outcomes, processes, or structures; analyzing and interpreting data; making and interpreting recommendations; monitoring and sustaining performance improvement.

    Examples:
    - Improved process for management of IV pumps
    - Redesign of nursing services orientation to increase satisfaction
    - Improved reimbursement for capsule endoscopy
    - Centers for Medicare & Medicaid Services core measures/quality indicators
    - 100,000 Lives Campaign
    - Joint Commission core measures: pregnancy and related conditions
    - National Patient Safety Goals
    - Quality scorecard

2. **Credentialed practitioners:** Verification and assessment; granting privileges based upon verification and assessment.

    Examples:
    - Physician credentialing process: receiving a request for an application, receiving a new application, verification process, completed application requirements
    - Preapplication form

Figure 10.7 (cont.)

Joint Commission leadership interview reference sheet

3. **Communication:** Process by which information is exchanged between individuals, departments, or organizations. Effective communication successfully permeates every aspect of a healthcare organization, from the provision of care to performance improvement, resulting in a marked improvement in the quality of care delivery and functioning.

   Examples:
   - Medication reconciliation process: medication reconciliation report changes, electronic documentation for capturing home medications, transfer information and discharge information to the patient
   - Implementation of Horizons Expert documentation: nursing plan of care, core measure documentation, medication reconciliation
   - Expansion of physician portal
   - Handoff processes (e.g., nurse to nurse, units to ancillary areas)
   - Rounding for outcomes

4. **Equipment use:** Equipment use incorporates the selection, delivery, setup, and maintenance of equipment and supplies to meet patient, client, resident, and staff needs. It generally includes movable equipment, as well as management of supplies that staff members use (e.g., gloves, syringes). Equipment use includes planning and selecting, maintaining, testing and inspecting, educating and providing instructions, delivery and setup, and risk prevention related to equipment/supplies.

   Examples:
   - Management plans for safety risks, hazardous materials and waste risks, emergency management, and fire-safety risks
   - Equipment preventive maintenance
   - Competencies in use of equipment required by job description
   - Maintaining clean and dirty linen rooms according to policy
   - References, books, periodicals, best practice (all known as "knowledge-based" information) are available through the hospital library, department-specific journals, and the Internet
   - Medications are secured at all times regardless of the location
   - Restraints are used infrequently and there is monitoring for compliance with policy

Figure 10.7 (cont.)

Joint Commission leadership interview reference sheet

- Resuscitation services are provided throughout the hospital; for example, by rapid response team
- Policy established to acquire, receive, store, and issue tissues; for example, in operating rooms

Clinical/service groups

Definition of clinical/service groups (CSGs)
Groups of patients in distinct clinical populations for which data are collected. Tracer patients are selected according to clinical service groups of high volume. For example:

1. Cardiology
2. General surgery
3. Vascular surgery
4. Gastroenterology
5. Orthopedic
6. Pulmonary

2006 National Patient Safety Goals (NPSGs)

1. Improve accuracy of patient identification
  a. Use of at least two patient identifiers
  b. "Time out" prior to procedure

2. Improve communication among caregivers
  a. Verbal order policy (RB/V)
  b. Unapproved abbreviations
  c. Timeliness of reporting critical lab and test results
  d. "Handoff" communications (when patient's caregiver changes)

3. Improve the safety of using medications
  a. Standardized drug concentrations
  b. Look-alike/sound-alike medications
  c. Labeling of medications and med containers

Figure 10.7 (cont.)

Joint Commission leadership interview reference sheet

4. Universal Protocol, wrong site procedure
    a. Preop checklist
    b. Site marking and "time out" prior to surgery

5. Reduce the risk of healthcare-associated infections
    a. Hand hygiene
    b. Review of sentinel events

6. Reconcile medications across the continuum of care
    a. Medication history upon admission
    b. Transfer/postprocedure report upon transfer
    c. Discharge medication report upon discharge

7. Reduce risk of injury related to falls
    a. Falls failure modes and effects analysis (FMEA) protocol

Failure modes and effects analysis

A failure modes and effects analysis (FMEA) is a comprehensive look at a process to determine
- where the error might occur
- how and why it might fail
- the effects if it does occur
- the probability of occurrence, detection, and severity
- actions to reduce the occurrence of the failure

Goals of an FMEA
- Be proactive to prevent failures from occurring
- Practice risk prevention
- Prevent errors and improve safety

Examples of FMEAs
- Patient falls, medication administration record verification, oxygen tanks, patient lifting, IV pole handling

Chapter 11

Case studies

This chapter provides a look at successful ongoing records review programs.

The first case study in this chapter demonstrates how Massachusetts General Hospital in Boston improved its ongoing records review process with the help of its physicians. The second highlights a new concept—Stop, Think, Act, Review, or STAR—to address legibility. The third—Memorial Health University Medical Center in Savannah, GA—shows how one hospital completely overhauled its records review process. The fourth—Port Huron Hospital in Port Huron, MI—developed a concurrent documentation review program.

The CD-ROM contains additional case studies that were previously published in the third edition of *Ongoing Records Review*. Greenville Hospital System, St. Vincent Hospital, and Roper Saint Francis Healthcare highlight methodologies you will find helpful as you work to meet The Joint Commission's new ongoing records review requirements. The other case studies—Antelope Valley Hospital; Crozer-Chester Medical Center; Holy Redeemer Hospital; and University of California, Irvine Medical Center—were developed before the 2004 standards. Although they do not reflect the 2004 standards, they represent good examples of the processes needed to develop and sustain a successful ongoing records review program.

Massachusetts General Hospital

A revamped process with physician support

When Marjorie Blundon, MBA, wanted to overhaul Massachusetts General Hospital's approach to ongoing records review last year, the health information services project specialist knew she had to win over at least one physician who could help her convince the entire medical staff that the plan would work if they would become involved in the process.

Chapter Eleven

Blundon was relatively new to the renowned Boston-based acute care hospital. She had only worked at the hospital for a year and a half, and with no clinical background, Blundon realized that she needed the support of a strong, well-respected clinician in the organization to make the change. She found her advocate to be—Gerald S. Foster, MD, a physician who initially opposed her plan.

Out with the old

Basically, Blundon wanted to expand the ongoing records review process from beyond the confines of the health information management (HIM) department to include the entire medical staff. The previous process left it up to HIM staff to handle the quarterly ongoing records reviews, which involved checking a small sampling of closed medical records on several inpatient units against the 19 elements listed under the old Joint Commission standard.

But because The Joint Commission's new ongoing records review requirement is less prescriptive and gives hospitals greater leeway in developing individual records review processes, Blundon thought the time was right to institute the new process. It also coincided with The Joint Commission's new survey approach to use the medical record and follow the patient's path, talking to the caregivers who provided care and treatment.

In with the new

To minimize the burden on one team made up of HIM staff and a few nurses, Blundon proposed creating five separate teams of 40 clinicians each to review records every two months on each of the hospital's 42 inpatient units. Each member would be responsible for reviewing three records twice a year, which would mean that at the end of each year the hospital would have reviewed 525 records.

Her proposal, however, met with much resistance. Every time Blundon mentioned it at a clinical policy and records committee meeting, Foster told her he didn't think it would work. "But I just kept coming back to the meetings, refining my ideas. Finally Dr. Foster said, 'You know, I think it might work,' and he agreed to sponsor it. He introduced me to all the physicians groups," Blundon said.

The two took their idea "on the road," explaining the concept at meetings and inviting clinical staff who document in patients' medical records to join the teams. They stressed the concept that the medical record reviews would lead to improving patient safety in documentation. "The medical record is the foundation for patient care and safety, so it only makes sense that it's accurate, complete, and timely," Blundon says.

Blundon then introduced a one-page, easy-to-use assessment form that listed all the items the team should review against the medical record (see Figure 11.1).

"I presented our idea and invited them to participate in the process. When I walked out of there, I went under the assumption they were doing it. I never asked them to actually sign up for it," she recalls.

Help with the process

She assigned each team member to a patient care unit, providing each with a range of room numbers to avoid duplication. Members had two weeks to complete three open records reviews by October 14, 2005. To keep the teams on track, Blundon sent a hospitalwide reminder via e-mail in August outlining what the teams needed to review, as well as follow-up e-mails in September that included their unit assignments and a copy of the data collection tool.

Each team member was asked to pull three medical records of patients currently admitted to the assigned unit and complete by hand the data collection tool for each of those records. To make it easier for physicians to complete, the sheet listed all the questions in a yes or no format. Once completed, the HIM staff entered the data into a spreadsheet created in Plato.

Report the results

Although not everyone participated in the actual process, and it took longer to complete than expected, Blundon was pleased with the results. One hundred and twenty people reviewed 334 records in four weeks. "I considered it a success," she says.

She then went back to the physicians groups to present her results, highlighting the main findings. Their weak areas: legible signatures and the use of unacceptable abbreviations in the medical record.

Because there was misinterpretation over the hospital's policy that physicians sign records using their "full signatures," the clinical policy and records committee clarified it to include language from the actual Joint Commission standard, which states that the records need to be authenticated by one of the following methods:

- Written, legible signature
- Rubber stamp signature
- Electronic signature

Chapter Eleven

Figure 11.1

Sample open record review form

Facility:	Medical record no.:
Admit date:	Review date:
Attending physician:	Service:
Patient care unit:	Reviewer:

Description	Patient Record Policy	Yes	No	N/A	Comments
PURPLE Tab (Admission/Discharge Information)					
Healthcare proxy (advance directives) or completed questionnaire present?	(3.1)				
ORANGE Tab (History & Physical/Progress Notes)					
Does the history contain chief complaint? details of present illness? relevant past, social, and family histories? inventory by body system?	(3.1)				
Summary of patient's psychosocial needs? (May be found in either MD or RN assessment notes)	(3.1)				
Report of relevant physical examination?	(3.1)				
Conclusions or impressions drawn from the admission H&P exam?	(3.1)				
Course of action planned for episode of care and its periodic review?	(3.1)				

136 © 2007 HCPro, Inc. ONGOING RECORDS REVIEW, FIFTH EDITION

CASE STUDIES

Figure 11.1 (cont.)

Sample open record review form

Description	Patient Record Policy	Yes	No	N/A	Comments
Admission note by attending physician?	(3.1)				
Nursing assessment?	(3.2.2)				
Is there a **daily** progress note by physician or designee for the past five days?	(3.4.1)				
Are all the progress notes dated for the past five days only? If NO, estimate % of compliance in Comments column	(3.4.1)				
Are all the progress notes signed with **full name** and **licensure** for the past five days? If NO, estimate % of compliance in Comments column	(3.4.1)				
If consult is present, is there a request or order? (If not in the chart, check POE)	(3.4.2)				
Brief op note entered immediately after surgery?	(3.3.3)				
YELLOW tab (Surgical/Invasive Procedures, Blood Transfusions)					
Evidence of informed consent?	(3.1)				
Evidence of an updated assessment note by responsible surgeon on day of procedure?	(3.3.2)				

Source: Massachusetts General Hospital. Reprinted with permission.

Chapter Eleven

In addition, the HIM staff created several new forms, including new day-of-surgery preprocedure note, brief operative report, and progress notes, that listed the unacceptable abbreviations in bold at the bottom of each page (see Figures 11.2, 11.3, and 11.4). "They felt it was a gentle reminder and less obtrusive way to remember them. Our compliance is much better now," she says.

Plans for the future

With the help of a small focus group, Blundon has improved the data classification with the form and has expanded the Plato physician table to drill down the records by subspecialty. She has also set up a sheet that provides team members with tips on three places to look for certain criteria.

Blundon intends to conduct the hospitalwide reviews quarterly, focusing on weaker areas that emerged from the previous ongoing records review. "For example, if we measure on 23 criteria and we do well on 13, I want to focus on the 10 areas of noncompliance to help improve those numbers," she says.

CASE STUDIES

Figure 11.2

Progress note

Enter name and unit number on both sides of EVERY sheet, Addressograph plate to be used when available. Name and unit number to be written distinctly when plate is not available.

Signature should be legible and include **full name, licensure and pager #**

DATE	TIME	

UNACCEPTABLE ABBREVIATIONS:	Applies to all handwritten and electronic 'free text' entries
QD QOD MS MSO$_4$ MgSO$_4$ hs ss µg U IU os qn bt	
.5 (i.e., use 0.5mg) 1.0 (i.e., use 1mg) Apothecary Symbols (e.g., amp, grain)	

Source: Massachusetts General Hospital. Reprinted with permission.

ONGOING RECORDS REVIEW, FIFTH EDITION © 2007 HCPro, Inc. **139**

Chapter Eleven

Figure 11.3

Brief operative report

Enter name and unit number on both sides of EVERY sheet, Addressograph plate to be used when available. Name and unit number to be written distinctly when plate is not available.

Signature should be legible and include **full name, licensure and pager #**

DATE	TIME	

Pre-op Diagnosis:

Post-op Diagnosis:

Procedure:

Surgeon:

Assistants:

Anesthesia:

Findings:

Specimens:

Complications:

Estimated Blood Loss:

IV Fluids:

Urinary Output:

Condition / Disposition:

Signature: _____, M.D.

UNACCEPTABLE ABBREVIATIONS: Applies to all handwritten and electronic 'free text' entries

| QD | QOD | MS | MSO$_4$ | MgSO$_4$ | hs | ss | µg | U | IU | os | qn | bt |

.5 (i.e., use 0.5mg)   1.0 (i.e., use 1mg)   Apothecary Symbols (e.g., amp, grain)

Source: Massachusetts General Hospital. Reprinted with permission.

Figure 11.4

Day-of-surgery preprocedure note

Enter name and unit number on both sides of EVERY sheet, Addressograph plate to be used when available. Name and unit number to be written distinctly when plate is not available.

Signature should be legible and include **full name, licensure and pager #**

DATE	TIME	Have there been any changes in the patient's health history obtained on:_____
		(check one) Yes:____ No:____
		If yes, please explain below:

Signature: _____, M.D.

UNACCEPTABLE ABBREVIATIONS: Applies to all handwritten and electronic 'free text' entries

| QD | QOD | MS | MSO$_4$ | MgSO$_4$ | hs | ss | µg | U | IU | os | qn | bt |

.5 (i.e., use 0.5mg)   1.0 (i.e., use 1mg)   Apothecary Symbols (e.g., amp, grain)

Source: Massachusetts General Hospital. Reprinted with permission.

CHAPTER ELEVEN

Using the STAR technique to improve legibility

One East Coast hospital successfully improved legibility of physicians' orders and notes by introducing the STAR technique to its medical staff.

The organization decided to try the technique in summer 2004, after Joint Commission surveyors cited the facility for illegible entries and it had to develop a corrective action plan to show how it planned to fix the problem. Through monitoring of illegible handwriting orders in the pharmacy, the organization had already identified the 13 physicians who were the biggest offenders.

The medical staff considered bringing in someone to teach a course on legibility, but decided against it because they had offered a similar program in the past and few physicians had attended. The medical staff were already familiar with the STAR technique (see Chapter 9 for more information) because The Greeley Company, a division of HCPro, had already introduced the concept in a general overview about skill-based, rule-based, and knowledge-based errors in an effort to improve behaviors in communication and patient safety.

Physicians held accountable

The simple STAR technique allows physicians to check their own writing: If they can't read the words they just wrote, then no one can, and they must correct the problem immediately. The president of the medical staff decided to use the technique in a more intensive way to get the problematic physicians to pay attention and slow down when writing orders.

To do so, the president of the medical staff gathered the data of the incidents of illegible orders and met individually with each of the primary offenders for 15–20 minutes to discuss the importance of legibility, compliance issues, and the STAR technique. The technique is based on the concept that illegible handwriting is the result of time pressure and heavy workload. That is, people are basically in a hurry when they write. STAR poses that anyone can write clearly if he or she slows down and pays more attention to what he or she is doing. It calls for physicians to stop for a second before they write orders, consider that the order needs to be written slowly enough to be legible, write the order slowly and legibly, and then review the order to make sure it can be read. If it's not legible, physicians must fix it right then. The medical staff leader had the physicians practice the simple technique in front of him.

To constantly remind physicians to slow down, the hospital had the words Stop, Think, Act, and Review printed at the bottom of all order sheets. For example, if physicians think that printing the orders rather than using a script style would help with legibility, then they are encouraged to use the STAR technique to remind themselves to print and to check that the printing is legible. The medical staff leader also reminded physicians to use the STAR technique when writing chart entries.

An ongoing process

Following the individual meetings, the organizations collected data on these physicians for two months and saw a dramatic increase in the number of legible orders. The hospital submitted the plan and the subsequent results to The Joint Commission, and the accreditor accepted it.

Since then, the organization has created a self-teaching module of the STAR technique. It includes a post-test that physicians must take at the time of reappointment or when issues arise over legibility. The post-test calls for physicians to practice writing an order set, review it for legibility, correct it if necessary, and pass in the test.

The medical staff also approved a legibility policy (see Figure 11.5) that is strictly enforced. Under this policy, physicians who have problems writing legible orders are monitored for two weeks. If there is improvement, the monitoring will continue for 90 days, and the physician will receive monthly feedback and discussion if the problem recurs. If illegibility is still an issue after the first two weeks, the proctor will meet with the individual physician to discuss the problem and reinforce the technique. If no improvement occurs after two more weeks, the medical staff would initiate the alternatives described in the policy.

Figure 11.5

Sample medical staff legibility policy

Purpose

In addition to the fact that it is a regulatory requirement receiving increased scrutiny, legibility of written orders is critical for effective communication among caregivers, for staff efficiency, and as a means of reducing the likelihood of medical errors. The legibility of physician orders and notes has long been problematic in the vast majority of hospitals using nonelectronic forms of physician documentation. As such, the medical staff is responsible for improving physician performance, both individually and aggregately, such that physician entries into the medical record can be read accurately by appropriate staff.

Figure 11.5 (cont.)

Sample medical staff legibility policy

Policy

To improve physician performance in this area, the medical staff has developed and approved the following policy and procedure.

Expectation

Physicians will use readable communication techniques when making entries into the medical record.

- Techniques for creating readable entries may include readable handwritten script or printing, transcribed dictations, computer-generated text documents, or direct computer entries.

- In generating the entries, the physician may personally make the chart entry, use the hospital or a personal transcription service where appropriate, or employ a scribe to generate the entry with the physician's signature and a legible identifier attesting to its accuracy.

- The definition of an unreadable entry is an entry that cannot be accurately and unambiguously interpreted by licensed professionals who are required to either act upon the entry or use the information in the entry for patient care and safety.

Performance measurement

Initial method

Based on a sample audit of charts for legibility over the past three months, physicians identified as having multiple occurrences of illegible entries will have the illegible entries validated by review of the medical staff president, VPMA, and MSQC chair. If the illegibility is substantially validated, the physician will be required to participate in performance management as described below.

Ongoing method

Upon approval of the MEC, the following method will be implemented to assess performance of all physicians on a routine basis:

- Indicator: Medication orders that cannot be accurately and unambiguously interpreted by the pharmacist and one additional licensed professional staff member (e.g., nurse, respiratory therapist, other physician) as appropriate to the unit, department, or specialty related to the patient's care

- Indicator type: Rule indicator

Figure 11.5 (cont.)

Sample medical staff legibility policy

- Indicator tracer population: All written medication orders submitted to pharmacy

- Indicator targets: Excellence: ≤ 4 unreadable orders per year;
  Acceptable: ≤ 12 unreadable orders per year

- Procedure:

    - Upon receiving a medication order that is unreadable, the entering pharmacist will contact the unit or department related to the order and request assistance with interpretation from a licensed professional caring for the patient.

    - If this individual cannot unambiguously interpret the order, the order will be deemed unreadable.

    - If the order is unreadable, by both the pharmacist and the caregiver, the pharmacist will contact the physician generating the order for clarification prior to filling the order. If the physician generating the order is not identifiable, the pharmacist will contact the attending of record or the covering physician for clarification. If the responding physician is uncooperative or verbally abusive to the pharmacist, the incident shall be reported to the medical staff president for follow-up.

- Data collection: A copy of all unreadable orders will be placed in a folder by the pharmacist and sent to the medical staff office at least monthly. The medical staff office will send out rule letters to the relevant physicians on a monthly basis and enter the data in the peer review database.

Performance feedback

The medical staff office will send out rule letters to the relevant physicians on a monthly basis and enter the data in the peer review database. If the number of incidents during any consecutive 12 months exceeds the acceptable target for the indicator, the individual orders for that period will be reviewed by the MSQC chair and two additional members to validate that all of the orders are illegible. If some of the orders are determined to be readable such that the target was not exceeded, the MSQC will send the physician a letter indicating the current total of illegible orders and reminding the physician of the acceptable target. If all of the orders are validated as illegible, the MSQC will inform the medical staff president.

Figure 11.5 (cont.)

Sample medical staff legibility policy

Performance management

The medical staff president will notify the physician by certified letter and a phone call to the physician's office that he or she must meet with the president, or if he or she is unavailable, with a medical staff officer designee, within two weeks of receiving the notice to begin the improvement process. The letter will also indicate the consequence for failure to meet, as described below.

The initial improvement process will be training in self-checking, which will be performed during the initial meeting with the medical staff president. Orders will be monitored for legibility over the next two weeks, and the physician will be provided with the results. If there is improvement (e.g., no more than one illegible order in the two-week period), the monitoring will continue for 90 days with semimonthly feedback. If more than four illegible orders are detected in the 90-day period, further discussion will be required.

If illegibility is still an issue after the first two weeks of monitoring, or if the problem returns during or after the monitoring period, the medical staff president or designee will meet with the physician again to discuss the problem and reinforce the technique. If no improvement is seen after an additional month, more rigorous alternatives will be initiated by the MEC based on the recommendations of the medical staff president to either restrict the physician's method for chart entry or restrict or remove the physician's membership or privileges. The board quality committee will be informed on a routine basis of the success rate for the training and the alternative measures used when training was not successful.

Corrective action

If the physician voluntarily accepts the above alternatives, no further action is needed. If not, the medical staff or the physician may pursue formal corrective action.

Failure to meet with the medical staff president to discuss the issue at any time during this process will result in an automatic suspension from the medical staff until the meeting occurs. The physician will be notified of the suspension by certified letter and a phone call to his of her office. The MEC, the hospital president, and the chair of the quality committee board will be informed of any such suspensions. Except for issues of disability or vacation, if the suspension lasts for 30 days, the failure to meet will be considered an automatic voluntary resignation from the medical staff. If the physician wishes to return to the staff, he or she will be required to go through the routine process for new applicants.

Memorial Health University Medical Center

New system saves times, improves value of collected data

A few years ago, ongoing records review was not going well for the Memorial Health University Medical Center in Savannah, GA.

Staff were using The Joint Commission's six-page records review tool—when they reviewed records at all—and using that method made each review take at least an hour to complete, according to Sherry Sweek, RHIA, CPHQ, outcomes and performance improvement coordinator. Closed record review meetings, held every two months, usually lasted longer than two hours.

"Medical records showed up with a stack of charts, and whoever came to the meeting reviewed them," she says. But there was no incentive for doing it and no mechanism by which to make people do it. "This was the last thing on the list for everybody," she says. In addition, the medical records staff conducted separate clinical pertinence reviews, which meant a lot of redundancy. It was a very non-user-friendly system, according to Sweek.

Start from a blank piece of paper

Sweek knew the process didn't work and had to be fixed. "We pretty much started from a blank piece of paper," she says. Sweek and her team interviewed staff to find out whether they performed records reviews and why or why not, what kind of data would be valuable to users, and what kind of feedback would be valuable to reviewers.

A major challenge for Sweek was turning a haphazard process into a timely system that helped departments take action to improve. Before, staff would turn in review forms, and the medical records department would enter data from a huge stack of paper. "We were lucky if we got a report eight months after the fact. There was never any feedback to anyone on how their department was doing," she says.

Knowing the existing problems and armed with the information gathered through staff interviews, Sweek and her team "knew we had to do something very basic and very easy. People want feedback and timely feedback," she says. "They want review questions that relate to their area and what they do. They want to be able to have a very easy, seamless process that doesn't take up a lot of time."

Simplifying and eliminating redundancy

First, Sweek looked at all 250 questions on The Joint Commission review form and determined which were appropriate for open review. "If a question relates to discharge, it doesn't make sense to have it on an open review," she explains. By combining clinical pertinence, Sweek reduced the reviews that the medical records department needed to conduct. Simplifying the forms was a priority. "Just because The Joint Commission asks a question that's 58 words long doesn't mean that we can't shorten it," says Sweek.

Another obstacle Sweek wanted to overcome was the question of how many records it's appropriate to review. "Everyone said the volume was too much, but we didn't know what it needed to be," she says. The final decision was 10 chart reviews per area per month. Before, people had turned in their reviews quarterly. Sweek also helped winnow down the review questions, resulting in six different one-page open records review forms:

1. Adult inpatient (see Figure 11.6)
2. Pediatrics
3. Emergency department
4. Psychiatry
5. Ambulatory care (e.g., family practice clinic, wound care, diabetes wellness center)
6. Operative and invasive (e.g., endoscopy, day surgery, PACU)

Each form has about 15 questions that directly apply to the unit's particular type of patients and that are answered "yes," "no," or "not applicable." Sweek eliminated from the forms topics that were not problematic. "We focused on problem areas like restraints, some of our operative data, and moderate sedation," she says. Each form begins with general questions, such as presence of general consent and a history and physical, and then moves on to more care-specific questions.

Figure 11.6

Sample open records review tool—adult inpatients

USE INK ONLY
Shade circles like this ●
Not like this ⊗ ☑

Y = Yes
N = No
S = N/A

Department
○ 3CSU   ○ CVICU
○ 4C   ○ GISU
○ 4ONC   ○ MOTHERBABY
○ 5C   ○ MSI
○ 5NS   ○ MST
○ 5VAS   ○ NEURO ICU
○ CCU   ○ OBS
○ ORTHO

Medical record number
[ ][ ][ ][ ][ ][ ][ ]

Date of teview (mm/dd/yy)
[ ][ ] [ ][ ] [ ][ ]

Admit date
[ ][ ] [ ][ ] [ ][ ]

GENERAL REVIEW/ASSESSMENTS: REVIEW ENTIRE CHART

Ⓨ Ⓝ Ⓐ Q3   General consent for treatment signed.
Ⓨ Ⓝ Ⓐ Q22   Record is legible. (Review progress notes, orders.)
Ⓨ Ⓝ Ⓐ Q150 Patient has an advance directive?
Ⓨ Ⓝ Ⓐ Q5   A copy if the advance directive is on the chart or the substance is documented in the medical record.
Ⓨ Ⓝ Ⓐ Q7   History and physical completed within 24 hours of admission. (May be dictated or handwritten. Must be within 30 days and updated.)
Ⓨ Ⓝ Ⓐ Q10   Admission database done within 12 hours of admit (nutrition, function, alcohol, abuse, safety, D/C planning).
Ⓨ Ⓝ Ⓐ Q145 Did database show additional assessments were needed?
Ⓨ Ⓝ Ⓐ Q12   Additional assessments completed within 24 hours. ○ Nutrition   ○ Function   ○ D/C plan   ○ Other
Ⓨ Ⓝ Ⓐ Q27   Verbal order/telephone orders documented as RB&V.
Ⓨ Ⓝ Ⓐ Q146 List unit(s) other than your unit where VO/TO not written as RB&V.
Ⓨ Ⓝ Ⓐ Q8   Pain is assessed at least every shift. (Review last 3 days only.)
Ⓨ Ⓝ Ⓐ Q131 If pain was present, intervention was done within 1 hour. (Mark **A** if patient did not have pain that required intervention.)

RESTRAINTS FOR MEDICAL/SURGICAL (Review last 3 days only)

Ⓨ Ⓝ Ⓐ Q79   An individual order is used for restraints.
Ⓨ Ⓝ Ⓐ Q133 Order for restraint is time limited and no greater than 24 hours.
Ⓨ Ⓝ Ⓐ Q80   Patient in restraints is monitored every 30 minutes.

OPERATIVE PROCEDURES (General Surgery only)

Ⓨ Ⓝ Ⓐ Q43   Risks, benefits, and alternatives are documented by physician in progress note, H&P, output H&P, MD office notes, or written in on consent form. CANNOT BE IN THE OP NOTE.
Ⓨ Ⓝ Ⓐ Q67   An operative note (handwritten) is on the chart immediately after surgery with **ALL** the following items: date, time, postop diagnosis, procedure, surgeon and assistants, estimated blood loss, and specimens removed.
Ⓨ Ⓝ Ⓐ Q148 Phase II recovery score completed. (Mark **A** if not recovering patient in your area.)
Ⓨ Ⓝ Ⓐ Q147 An anesthesia postop note (within 48 hours of surgery) is documented. (May be on anesthesia progress note.)

MODERATE SEDATION (Complete only if moderate sedation is given)

Ⓨ Ⓝ Ⓐ Q48   Patient is reevaluated immediately before moderate sedation by physician, and physician preprocedure note completed in full. (Mark **N** if there are any blanks.)
Ⓨ Ⓝ Ⓐ Q149 Phase II recovery score completed. (Mark **A** if not recovering patient in your area.)
Ⓨ Ⓝ Ⓐ Q143 Was a reversal agent used?

Reviewer name: _____

Complete 10 charts per month. Due by 15th of next month.
Please return to: HIM

Source: Memorial Health University Medical Center, Savannah, GA. Reprinted with permission.

Chapter Eleven

Timeliness, compliance, and meaning

Because the medical records department receives and scans the forms into an access database, Sweek can create customized reports for each area of the hospital. Each unit can go into an internal Web site, aggregate its data, and compare its unit to the rest of the hospital. The department trends over the past four quarters are available, as well. "It's all electronic. We don't print out any reports for a unit," Sweek says. Figures below The Joint Commission threshold are in red on the online version and in bold on a printed report.

The other benefit of this system is its timeliness. "I can scan some reviews in today and query some data this afternoon," she says. The facility is also getting information from cases it was never able to review. "Before, we never got any information back on longer-term patients. Staff said it would take too long to get through the chart." However, she decided that because documentation is generally either really good or really bad, it doesn't take a 10-day review to determine that. Therefore, reviewers now review a snapshot of the longer records from the past three or five days.

Sweek now boasts 98% compliance overall for reviews. The time for a nurse to review a chart concurrently is about 10 minutes, instead of an hour. "On a quarterly basis, we usually have 200–300 responses, so the data is a good volume of what we do," she says. By cutting through the time it took just to conduct the reviews and aggregate the data, Sweek and her team now have time to analyze the data, find issues, and fix problems. "We can do timely interventions," she says.

Sweek receives positive responses about this system from everyone who participates in it or has seen how it works, she reports. "We feel pretty good about it. I think that we're doing a lot more reviews than other hospitals, and they're more meaningful. When there is an issue, we're doing something to address it, and we're providing data so units can take action. I think that's been extremely helpful."

Allow for ongoing modification

The automated ongoing records review system went through the pilot phase in the fourth quarter of 2002. Sweek asked five areas to use the form she created and provide feedback. They made modifications based on the feedback.

"We figured out our process and put it all down in writing so we could share it with people," says Sweek. Sharing involved attending committee meetings and providing inservices. The process went live in January 2003.

Sweek wanted to be able to modify forms along the way. "Let's say there are two new Joint Commission standards that come out that are very problematic. We want to be able to start collecting data on that in a timely manner."

For example, the state of Georgia changed its rules and regulations to say that if the verbal order is written, repeated, and verified, then the order can be signed within 30 days after discharge with the rest of the record.

"We wanted to start tracking our areas to see if they're writing the verbal and doing the repeat and verify, so we started collecting that information."

Saving time, improving results

Closed records review meetings are still held every other month, but they now last 30–45 minutes at the most. The six-page form was cut down to two pages by limiting questions to only those that apply at discharge. Reviews that routinely took more than an hour before now take 20 minutes at the most. The medical records department assigns reviews. Everyone receives three charts to review before the meeting. Reviewers turn in their forms prior to the meeting so medical records staff can aggregate the data.

"We're talking about real-time data," says Sweek. "We use the meeting to discuss whether we're finding something on closed reviews very problematic that we should put on the open review." Also, if something is not a problem, the closed records review committee may decide to remove it from the review form.

Port Huron Hospital

Accountability is the foundation of a successful concurrent documentation review process for 186-bed Port Huron Hospital, in Port Huron, MI.

Several years ago, the facility had a closed medical records review in which a multidisciplinary team reviewed records monthly, says Lynn Frazer, medical records data analyst. By 2002, however, it had moved to half closed and half open records reviews. But documentation deficiencies were still an overriding struggle. Now, after developing the concurrent documentation review program, the facility can boast impressive improvements.

Chapter Eleven

For example, the incidence of RNs signing off on their documentation with signatures is now at 98%. History and physicals on the chart prior to a procedure has increased to 99%. Physician documentation of informed consent is now at 99%.

Regular review reports

The departments' commitment to documentation accountability led them to this success, says JoAnne Osterland, BS, RHIT, HIM supervisor for the hospital. Each unit has a designated quality assurance (QA) staff member who distributes 20 review forms a month to each unit, which works out to about five per nurse. Those QA staff members must conduct concurrent chart audits using the forms on the day they receive them. The QA staff member who distributed the forms then generates a monthly report based on the information in them.

The report is used for education during monthly staff meetings and process management meetings. The HIM department generates quarterly reports and presents "unit-specific" and "units overall" reports to the quality management committee and nursing leadership each quarter.

Each documentation-deficient chart gets a documentation quality accountability letter (see Figure 11.12 for a sample letter). This letter is forwarded by the QA nurse to any staff member who needs to complete missing documentation. If the record is still on the unit, the documentation is added right away. If the chart has reached discharged status, the nurse must go to the medical records department to complete the record. Once the documentation is complete, the nurse has his or her manager authenticate the accountability letter. All review forms are placed in nursing staff personnel files and used for the documentation portion of their yearly evaluations.

"It's all about accountability," says Frazer. "Because the nursing staff know that their documentation is being looked at, they're more apt to make sure they do the right thing first." And regularly conducting reviews ensures that documentation criteria are embedded in their thought processes so they automatically do it right the first time.

Results exceed needs

This process arose from a need to move from closed records review to open review, find a process that really worked, and figure out a way to use collected data. The process management team prepares a monthly report based on all of the chart reviews.

Case studies

The QA nurse uses a tally sheet (see Figure 11.7) that serves as a basis for improvement recommendations. The QA nurse may conduct one-on-one discussions with individual staff for education of identified documentation deficiencies. After presentations during the monthly staff meetings, the findings are posted on boards in each unit for viewing.

"We have everything documented as far as when we find the problem and how we fix it," says Frazer.

But Port Huron Hospital has experienced benefits far beyond what it had hoped. "One of the best successes of this process has been that we don't spend all of our time reviewing charts at these meetings," says Osterland. "We're actually hammering out any problems that they have from one unit to another in some of the documentation in the charts they're receiving from each other." The lines of communication have opened up, as well. "The outpatient clinics weren't originally part of this process, but they asked to become part of the regular monthly team so that they can share in the same information and get the advantage of communicating."

Chapter Eleven

Figure 11.7

Ongoing documentation review tally sheet—Second quarter, 2005

Monthly percentages			
Unit:	April # ___	May # ___	June # ___
Admission assessment			
Is the admission assessment completed and signed by RN? (No blanks or lines through any sections)			
Advance directive (AD)			
Was AD addressed on the admission assessment?			
Is the AD on the record? If not, is there documentation that family was asked to bring it to the hospital?			
Is there a physician order for code status?			
Nutrition screen			
If application, has a dietary consult been initiated?			
Pain			
When pain is identified, is an assessment is performed and documented?			
If pain medication is administered, is there a reassessment of the patient's pain level?			
Is regular reassessment of pain documented according to nursing policy, appropriate to patient's age/abilities?			
As appropriate to the patient's condition, is there documentation that the patient is educated about pain and methods for effective pain management?			
Procedures (any invasive procedure completed bedside)			
Is a valid history and physical (H&P) or consult present and updated within 24 hours of procedure start?			
Timed and dated? Postop progress note written by the physician immediately following all procedures?			
Universal Protocol form completed, signed, dated, and timed by the physician?			
Physician orders			
Are all of the orders signed off on by RNs? (Check for readable, dated, timed, prohibited abbreviations)			

Figure 11.7 (cont.)

Ongoing documentation review tally sheet—Second quarter, 2005

Monthly percentages			
Unit:	April # ___	May # ___	June # ___
Education/patient response			
Is there documentation of the patient's current medication regimen, including the patient's own perception of its effectiveness? Including first-dose effect?			
Was smoking counseling documented regarding tobacco use? (Current tobacco use within the past year.)			
Plan of care			
Nursing plan of care has been initiated and individualized for the patient and documented on admission.			
Nursing plan of care evaluative statement has been documented every shift.			
Heart failure (HF) only (Concurrent core measure review)			
HF clinical pathway initiated?			
HF ACE inhibitor prescribed if: EF < 40% and no contraindications documented?			
Pediatrics only			
Head circumference documented?			
Actual weight documented?			
Actual length/height documented?			
Current immunization status documented?			
Are patient's education needs addressed (if appropriate)?			
Mental health unit (MHU) only			
Psychiatric evaluation and H&P completed within 24 hours of admission? (If not, please indicate responsible physician.)			
Initial vital signs taken and documented?			
Does nursing (MHU) assessment include: history of emotional, behavioral, substance abuse problem; occurrence; and treatment?			
Does nursing (MHU) assessment include: current emotional and behavioral functioning and psychosocial assessment?			

CHAPTER ELEVEN

Figure 11.7 (cont.)

Ongoing documentation review tally sheet—Second quarter, 2005

Monthly percentages			
Unit:	April # ___	May # ___	June # ___
Interdisciplinary treatment plan done within 24 hours of admission and contains physician signature?			
Psychotropic med consent completed prior to starting any psychotropics?			
Family contract/meeting is done within 24 hours of admission?			
Activity therapy initial assessment done?			
Group therapy notes for all group sessions completed on the day session is held?			
Legal assessment, forms attached, when appropriate?			
Procedures (any invasive procedure done in OR setting)			
H&P on chart prior to procedure: Must be dictated within 30 days of procedure date; if H&P dictated more than 24 hours prior to procedure, it must be authenticated (signed, dated, timed) and updated with any changes in the patient's condition by the physician performing the procedure. This must be done prior to the start time of the procedure.			
All H&Ps dictated by PAs must be reviewed and cosigned by the surgeon prior to the start of procedure.			
Preanesthesia assessment documented prior to induction of anesthesia (contains anesthesiologist signature or initials)?			
Postanesthesia assessment completed/authenticated by anesthesiologist?			
Timed and dated? Postop progress note written by the physician immediately following all procedures?			
Universal Protocol form completed, signed, dated, and timed by the physician?			

Source: Port Huron Hospital, Port Huron, MI. Reprinted with permission.

Ready for anything

New or updated standards are easily thrown into the review mix. "We're already compliant with the 2004 patient safety standards by rolling the prohibited abbreviations list into our open record review process," says Frazer. Port Huron's process "makes the new Joint Commission IM standards flow a lot easier because they are reviewed in every area by the person who's actually the author of the documentation in the record."

Port Huron Hospital has joined the Michigan Hospital Association, the state's coordinating body, to work with the continual survey readiness program offered by Joint Commission Resources. Through that program, the hospital has already completed numerous patient tracers.

"We were one of the first organizations in Michigan to complete a periodic performance review," says Ronnie Walker, RN, BA, CHC, compliance officer and The Joint Commission director for the facility. "Prior to that, we did several tracers in order to verify that we were in compliance with the standards and the elements of performance to make sure that our measures of success were appropriate. We have found the documentation procedure to be extremely helpful in making sure that when we drill down, we actually have hard data, as opposed to people who said they did it but have no quantifiable methods with which to prove that."

Walker is pleased with the HIM department's efforts. "It's not been an overnight success. They've been working on this for a long time." As The Joint Commission person directing this effort, Walker is pleased about how thorough the data is. "This is no longer simply data. Through HIM's efforts, we have made it meaningful."

During Port Huron's Joint Commission survey in 2002, when it was doing about half closed and half open records reviews, the surveyors were already impressed with the process it had started and the direction in which it was headed, says Frazer.

The facility knew from the past that everyone geared up for The Joint Commission survey, but there were gaps, and there was very little time to manage those gaps before survey time. "There was always a hole that never allowed the data to go beyond being reported," says Osterland. "We realized that we needed to close that gap, and that wasn't going to happen without an accountability factor." Including the results of these documentation reviews in each employee's yearly evaluation helped get the buy-in from the personnel.

Chapter Eleven

"We've been very clear on that from a corporate compliance perspective and in our annual mandatory training," says Walker. "We petition every person who touches the chart in any way to ensure that the documentation is accurate, complete, and legible. That sounds like 'Documentation 101,' but it's amazing how many people find that to be somewhat new."

What this effort really illustrates is the partnership between accreditation and regulation and what its effect is on quality. Everyone works together "to do what's best for the patient," Walker says.

Osterland says the nurses have taken a real ownership in the process. "If we come up with a problem in documentation, they're the first ones to address it," she says. "They love it. Their records look better. The mindset used to be that documentation is a medical records problem. Now we're in the mindset that documentation is everyone's function."

Figures 11.8–11.12 illustrate other tools used by Port Huron Hospital to improve its ongoing records review.

Figure 11.8

Ongoing documentation review—Second quarter, 2005

MR#	Location of documentation:	Reviewer:		
Admission date:	Admission assessment/Horizon	Y	N	N/A
Admission assessment				
Is the admission assessment completed and signed by RN? (No blanks or lines through any sections)				
Advance directive (AD)				
Was AD addressed on the admission assessment?	Admission assessment			
Is the AD on the record? If not, is there documentation that family was asked to bring it to the hospital?	Check record for documentation			
Is there a physician order for code status?	Physician orders			
Nutrition screen				
If application, has a dietary consult been initiated?	Progress notes/teaching record/Horizon			
Pain				
When pain is identified, is an assessment performed and documented?	Flow sheets, Horizon, assessments			
If pain medication is administered, is there a reassessment of the patient's pain level?	Care plan, Horizon, teaching record			
Is regular reassessment of pain documented according to nursing policy, appropriate to patient's age/abilities?	Care plan, Horizon, teaching record			
As appropriate to the patient's condition, is there documentation that the patient is educated about pain and methods for effective pain management?	Care plan, Horizon, teaching record			
Procedures (any invasive procedure completed bedside)				
Valid history and physical (H&P) or consult present and updated within 24 hours of procedure start?	Check record for physician-updated H&P dictation or shortform			
Timed and dated? Postop progress note written by the physician immediately following all procedures?	Check progress notes			
Universal Protocol form completed, signed, dated, and timed by the physician?	Verify form			
Physicians orders				
Are all of the orders signed off on by RNs? (Check for readable, dated, timed, prohibited abbreviations.)	Physician orders			

CHAPTER ELEVEN

Figure 11.8 (cont.)

Ongoing documentation review—Second quarter, 2005

MR#	Location of documentation:	Reviewer:		
Admission date:	Admission assessment/Horizon	Y	N	N/A
Admission assessment				
Education/patient response				
Is there documentation of the patient's current medication regimen, including the patient's own perception of its effectiveness? Including first-dose effect?	Horizon, teaching record/progress notes/flow sheets/care plans			
Was smoking counseling documented regarding tobacco use? (Current tobacco use within the past year)	Horizon, teaching record/progress notes/flow sheets/care plans			
Plan of care				
Nursing plan of care has been initiated and individualized for the patient, and documented on admission?	Horizon, teaching record, STAR/profiles			
Nursing plan of care evaluative statement has been documented every shift?	Horizon, teaching record, STAR/profiles			
Heart failure (HF) only (Concurrent core measure review)				
HF clinical pathway initiated?	Horizon, teaching record/progress notes/flow sheets/care plans			
HF ACE inhibitor prescribed if: EF < 40% and no contraindications documented?	Physician orders, MAR sheets, care manager, reaching record			
Pediatrics only				
Head circumference documented?	Admission assessment/Horizon			
Actual weight documented?	Admission assessment/Horizon			
Actual length/height documented?	Admission assessment/Horizon			
Current immunization status documented?	Admission assessment/Horizon			
Are patient's education needs addressed (if appropriate)?	Admission assessment/Horizon/progress notes			
Mental health unit (MHU) only				
Psychiatric evaluation and H&P completed within 24 hours of admission? (If not, please indicate responsible physician.)	Check for dictation			

Figure 11.8 (cont.)

Ongoing documentation review—Second quarter, 2005

MR#	Location of documentation:	Reviewer:		
Admission date:	Admission assessment/Horizon	Y	N	N/A
Admission assessment				
Initial vital signs taken and documented?	Admission assessment			
Does nursing (MHU) assessment include: history of emotional, behavioral, substance abuse problem; occurrence; and treatment?	Admission assessment			
Does nursing (MHU) assessment include: current emotional and behavioral functioning and psychosocial assessment? Interdisciplinary treatment plan done within 24 hours of admission and contains physician signature?	Admission assessment			
Psychotropic med consent completed prior to starting any psychotropics?	Check for form on record			
Family contract/meeting is done within 24 hours of admission?	Check for form on record			
Activity therapy initial assessment done?	Check for form on record			
Group therapy notes for all group sessions completed on the day session is held?	Check for form on record			
Legal assessment, forms attached, when appropriate?	Check for form on record			
Procedures (any invasive procedure done in OR setting)				
H&P on chart prior to procedure: Must be dictated within 30 days of procedure date; if H&P dictated more than 24 hours prior to procedure, it must be authenticated (signed, dated, timed) and updated with any changes in the patient's condition by the physician performing the procedure. This must be done prior to the start time of the procedure.	Handwritten or dictated documentation			
All H&Ps dictated by PAs must be reviewed and cosigned by the surgeon prior to the start of procedure.	Handwritten or dictated documentation			
Preanesthesia assessment documented prior to induction of anesthesia (contains anesthesiologist signature or initials)?	Box at top of red anesthesia form or on procedure forms			
Postanesthesia assessment completed/authenticated by anesthesiologist?	Box on back of red anesthesia form or on procedure forms			
Timed and dated? Postop progress note written by the physician immediately following all procedures?	Progress notes			
Universal Protocol form completed, signed, dated, and timed by the physician?	Verify universal protocol form			

Source: Port Huron Hospital, Port Huron, MI. Reprinted with permission.

Chapter Eleven

Figure 11.9

Prohibited abbreviation documentation monitor

Reviewer: _____ Date: _____

Please indicate where found, who was responsible for documentation of prohibited abbreviation, whether you contacted that person, and whether correction was made.

Prohibited abbreviation	Physician	Nursing	Other discipline	Writer notified Y or N
U				
IU				
QD, Q.O.D				
Trailing zero (X.0 mg)				
Lack of leading zero (.X mg)				
MS, MSO$_4$, MgSO$_4$				
µg				
T.I.W.				
A.S., A.D., A.U.				
O.S., O.U.				

Comments

Source: Port Huron Hospital, Port Huron, MI. Reprinted with permission.

Figure 11.10

Prohibited abbreviation documentation tally

Month: _____ Unit: _____

Please specify how many of each of the prohibited abbreviations were found this month during your ongoing documentation reviews.

Prohibited abbreviation	Physician	Nursing	Other discipline	Total # found
U				
IU				
QD, Q.O.D				
Trailing zero (X.0 mg)				
Lack of leading zero (.X mg)				
MS, MSO$_4$, MgSO$_4$				
μg				
T.I.W.				
A.S., A.D., A.U.				
O.S., O.U.				

Comments

Action

Source: Port Huron Hospital, Port Huron, MI. Reprinted with permission.

CHAPTER ELEVEN

Figure 11.11

Action plan

Plans for improvement:		
Findings reported at staff meetings: (Dates)		
Results posted: (Dates)		
Provided 1:1 staff discussions		

Source: Port Huron Hospital, Port Huron, MI. Reprinted with permission.

CASE STUDIES

Figure 11.12

Accountability letter

Date: _____   Admit date: _____
Unit: _____   Discharge date: _____
To: _____

On _____, you were responsible for documentation on patient MR#_____.
The following required documentation components were not completed. As you know, the Joint Commission on Accreditation of Healthcare Organizations and Port Huron Hospital have stringent guidelines pertaining to documentation.

Please sign and return this letter to me upon completion of the documentation below:

❏ Admission assessment
❏ Advance directive/code status
❏ Nutrition screen/dietary consult initiated
❏ Pain documentation
❏ Physician orders
❏ Procedures (invasive bedside)
❏ Education/patient response
❏ Plan of care documentation
❏ Heart failure documentation
❏ Procedures (OR setting)
❏ Prohibited abbreviations: Used:
                              Location:
❏ Pediatrics
❏ Mental health
Comments:

Date completed:
Nurse signature:

      Thank you for contributing to the excellent care that we provide,

      Nursing leadership

Source: Port Huron Hospital, Port Huron, MI. Reprinted with permission.

CHAPTER 12

Sample review tools and reports

Figure 12.1

Respiratory therapy chart review tool

(Patient label)

Items reviewed P= presence A= absence N/A= not applicable	P or A	N/A	Comments
Initial orders			
Orders signed off on by therapist			
Documentation of the interdisciplinary plan of care			
1. Done by therapist doing initial treatment			
2. Date and time indicated			
3. Respiratory problems indicated			
4. Goals indicated related to problems			
5. Target time			
6. Interventions noted			
Interdisciplinary patient education			
1. Patient education noted on initial treatment			
2. Patient education noted with any change in respiratory therapy orders			
3. Patient education noted if related to family			
Interdisciplinary notes			
1. Treatments charted on either treatment or shift summary			
2. Indication of improvement post treatments			
3. Initials following notes			
4. Therapist signature and title			
Respiratory therapy treatment box			
1. Type of therapy box checked			
2. Frequency indicated			
3. Medication indicated			
4. Boxes initialed that indicate time of Tx			

Reviewer: _____   Date: _____

Figure 12.2

Medical records documentation audit tool—physician office

Physician: _____
Reviewer: _____
Date: _____

CHART ORDER/PERSONAL DATA/CONSENTS			
ITEM	YES	NO	COMMENTS
Appropriate chart order			
Name			
Address/home phone			
Employer/work phone			
Date of birth			
Marital status			
Emergency contact			
Sex			
Medical/family history			
Any impairments noted: hearing, speech, etc.			
Allergies noted			
Consent to treatment/procedures			
Medical diagnosis present			
Summary list initiated if appropriate			
DOCUMENTED EACH VISIT			
Chief complaint/reason for visit			
Physical exam findings			
Previous problem follow-up if appropriate			
Current medications			
Treatment plan			
Treatment documented			
Summary list updated			
Patient education regarding diet, meds, activities, return visit			
Patient ID on each page			
Entries legible and dated			
CONSULTATION, LAB, RADIOLOGY, OPERATIVE REPORTS, IMMUNIZATIONS, OTHER			
Reports on chart and initialed by appropriate caregiver			
Follow-up documented of abnormal test results			
Immunizations: Adult: Tetanus diphtheria booster			
Pediatrics: Immunization record			
Pediatrics: Growth chart			

Figure 12.3

Ongoing records review—inpatient records

MR #: **Date of service:**

Topic	Instructions	Yes	No	N/A	Dept/Unit	Physician responsible
Advance directives	Face sheet marked					
	Form on chart and complete, matches face sheet					
	Advance directive on chart if appropriate					
Consent to surgery	Before surgery					
	Signed by the MD					
History & physical	Documented within 24 hrs. after admission					
	Before surgery					
Postop progress note	Written immediately after surgery					
	Contains: procedure(s) surgeon and assistants; specimen(s) removed; complications, if any					
Operative report	Charted within 24 hrs. of surgery					
	Signed by MD					

Figure 12.4

Ongoing records review

Topic	Instructions	Yes	No	N/A	Physician responsible
Advance directives	Face sheet marked				
	Form on chart and complete, matches face sheet				
	Advance directive on chart if appropriate				
Informed consent	Before surgery				
	Signed by the MD				
History & physical	Documented within 24 hrs. after admission				
	Before surgery				
Postop progress note	Written immediately after surgery				
	Contains: procedure(s) surgeon and assistants; specimen(s) removed; complications, if any				
Operative report	Charted within 24 hrs. of surgery				
Initial nursing assessment	Signed by MD within 24 hrs.				
Pain assessment	Initial				
	Reassessed				
Screens	Nutritional				
	Functional				
	Discharge planning				
Response to screening referrals	Nutritional				
	Functional				
	Discharge planning				

Instructions:
1. Complete one for each chart
2. Leave form on the medical record at discharge
3. Indicate responsible physician in the areas that are not shaded

SAMPLE REVIEW TOOLS AND REPORTS

Figure 12.5

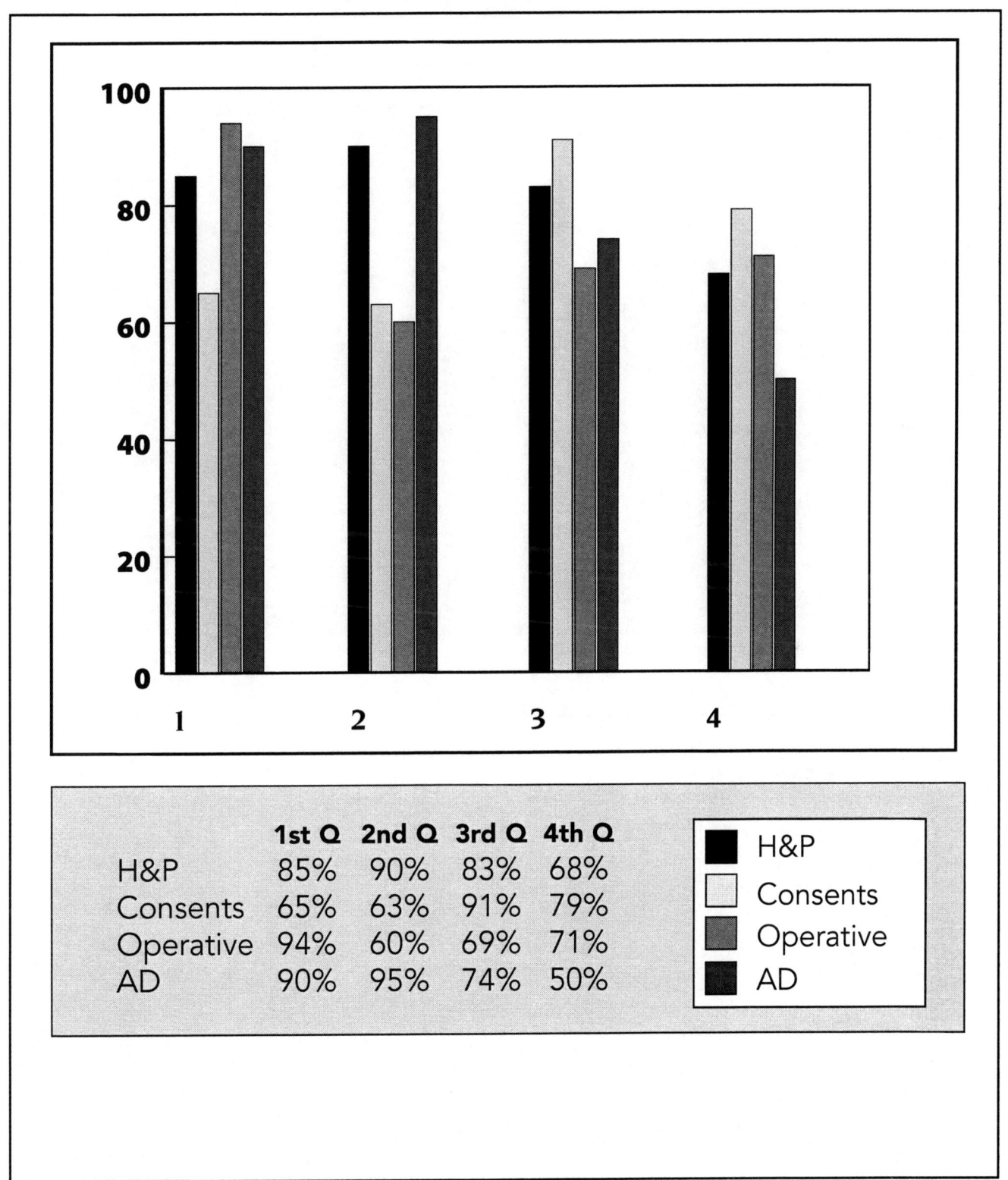

Ongoing records review graph

	1st Q	2nd Q	3rd Q	4th Q
H&P	85%	90%	83%	68%
Consents	65%	63%	91%	79%
Operative	94%	60%	69%	71%
AD	90%	95%	74%	50%

Legend: H&P, Consents, Operative, AD

ONGOING RECORDS REVIEW, FIFTH EDITION © 2007 HCPro, Inc. **173**

CHAPTER TWELVE

Figure 12.6

Medical record deficiency trend compared to monthly discharges

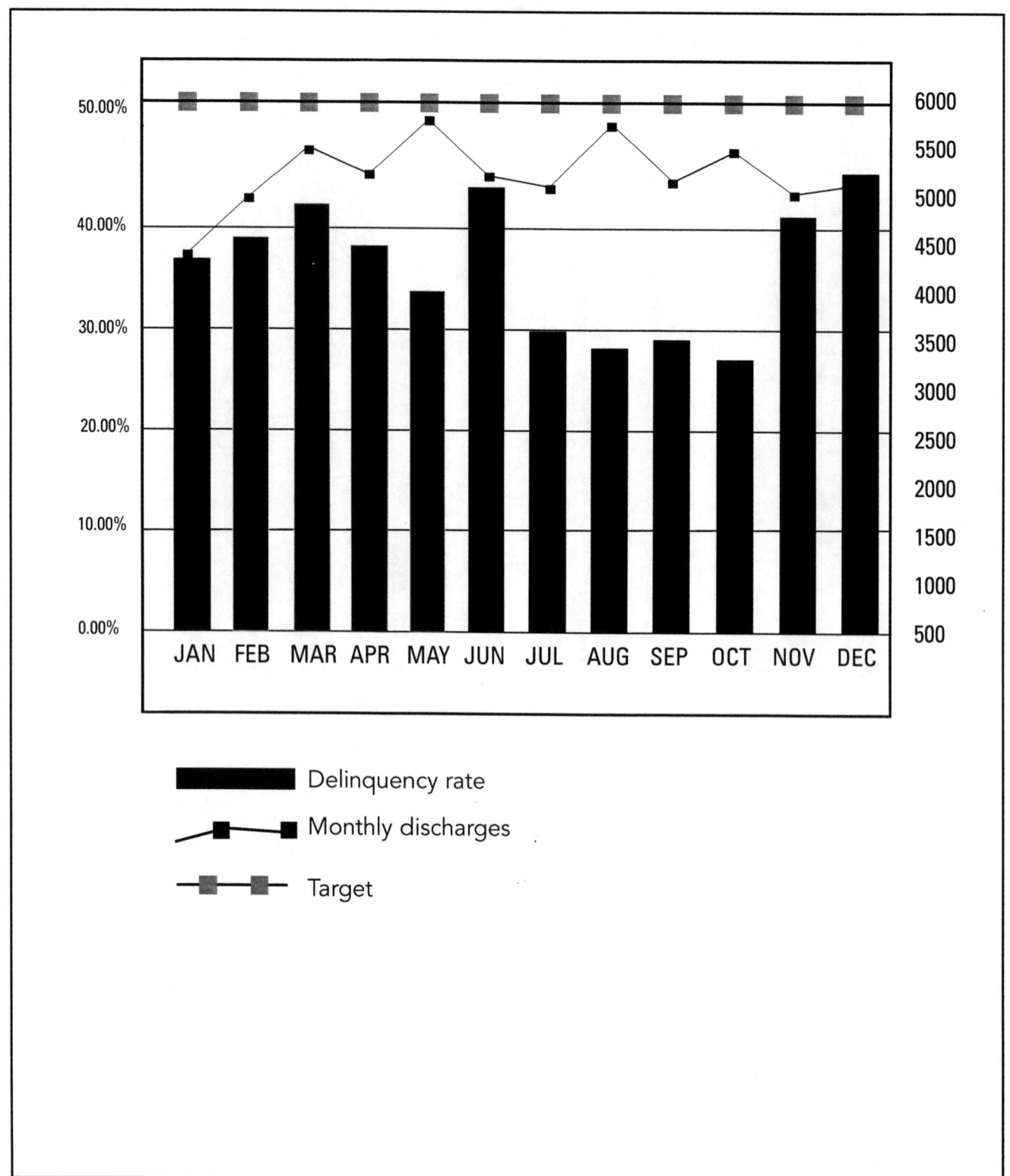

Figure 12.7

First and second quarter comparison: Ongoing records review percentage met

Compliance Rate - 1st Quarter n=280	Indicator	Hospital A n=150	Hospital B n=40	Hospital C n=90
99%	Medical History, including	97%	100%	100%
100%	Summary of the patient's psychosocial needs as appropriate to the patient's age	100%	100%	100%
99%	Report of relevant physical examinations	98%	100%	100%
98%	Statement on the conclusions or impressions drawn from the admission H&P exam	97%	97%	100%
99%	Statement on the course of action planned for this episode of care and its periodic review, as appropriate	99%	98%	100%
99%	Diagnostic and therapeutic orders	97%	100%	100%
93%	Evidence of appropriate informed consent	89%	95%	95%
100%	Clinical observations, including the results of therapy	100%	100%	100%
100%	Progress notes made by the medical staff and other authorized staff	100%	100%	100%
100%	Consultation reports if applicable	100%	100%	100%
99%	Reports of operative and other invasive procedures, tests, and their results if appropriate	99%	100%	99%
100%	Reports of any diagnostic and therapeutic procedures such as pathology and clinical laboratory examinations and radiology and nuclear medicine examinations or treatments	100%	100%	100%
99% n=233	Records of donation and receipt of transplants or implants if applicable	100% n=199	97% n=4	100% n=30
87%	Final diagnosis	88%	80%	94%
98%	Conclusions at termination of hospitalization	95%	98%	100%
98%	Clinical resumes and discharge summaries	95%	100%	100%
86%	Discharge instructions to pt and/or family	95%	62%	100%
100%	Results of autopsy, when performed	100% n=6	100% n=4	100% n=4

CHAPTER TWELVE

Figure 12.8

Quarterly review summary

Quarterly Summary Report

Topic	1st Quarter	2nd Quarter	3rd Quarter	4th Quarter
AD	50%	76%	55%	18%
Consent to Tx, signed	71%	70%	61%	82%
VO/48 hrs., signed	72%	71%	85%	60%
Entries according to policy signed	58%	58%	70%	47%
Treatment plans	94%	95%	100%	87%
H&P/24 hrs.	68%	75%	65%	65%
Nursing assessment	98%	98%	100%	97%
Learning needs	99%	94%	100%	97%
Nutritional assessment	94%	87%	100%	96%
Functional assessment	90%	83%	90%	94%
Discharge planning A	92%	92%	90%	95%
Developmental age (peds)	95%	94%	95%	
Reassessed	99%	98%	100%	99%
Informed consent, signed	79%	38%	100%	98%
Preanesthesia assessment	95%	90%	100%	98%
Preop plan for anesthesia	88%	89%	80%	96%
Nursing care plan	94%	83%	100%	98%
Anesthesia reevaluation	87%	86%	80%	94%
Physiological assess	89%	89%	80%	98%
Op report dictated	71%	88%	80%	46%
Postoperative PN	80%	75%	80%	86%
Signed op report	63%	84%	60%	44%
PACU monitoring	96%	93%	100%	96%
PACU discharged by criteria/MD signature	94%	85%	100%	96%
Ambulatory summary	98%	100%		96%
Emergency dept.				
• Care prior to arrival	94%	95%	100%	87%
• Conclusions	43%	43%	100%	100%
• Transfers	99%	99%	100%	13%
Restraints				
• Order	53%	77%	83%	0%
• Time limited	78%	85%	83%	67%
• Justification	81%	77%	100%	67%

Figure 12.9
Ongoing records review—closed charts, discharge summary content

Topic: Discharge summary
(Consider the following when reviewing the discharge summary and its content: presence, timeliness, quality, readability, consistency, clarity, accuracy, completeness, and authentication.)
√ indicates YES. X indicates NO

Information/Indicator	MR#	MR#	MR#	MR#	MR#	MR#	MR#
1. MD							
2. Discharge date							
3. Is the DS on the chart (or electronically available) within 30 days of discharge?							
4. Does the DS contain:							
4a. Reason for hospitalization							
4b. Significant findings							
4c. Procedures and care, treatment, and services provided							
4d. Patient's condition at discharge							
4e. Instructions to patient and family, as appropriate?							
5. Is the DS readable and free of blanks?							
6. Does the DS contain abbreviations from the prohibited list?							
7. Is the DS authenticated?							
8. Comments							

9. Action needed?	What	Who	When due